Craniofacial and Dental Developmental Defects

J. Timothy Wright

Editor

Craniofacial and Dental Developmental Defects

Diagnosis and Management

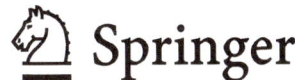 Springer

Editor
J. Timothy Wright
Department of Pediatric Dentistry
University of North Carolina
School of Dentistry
Chapel Hill, NC
USA

ISBN 978-3-319-34531-4   ISBN 978-3-319-13057-6   (eBook)
DOI 10.1007/978-3-319-13057-6
Springer Cham Heidelberg New York Dordrecht London

Printed on acid-free paper

Springer is part of Springer Science+Business Media (www.springer.com)

Contents

Developmental Defects of the Craniofacial Complex and Dentition: Scope and Challenges

1

J. Timothy Wright

Abstract

Providers of oral health care are faced with rapid changes in knowledge related to the etiology, diagnosis, and treatment of conditions affecting the oral and craniofacial health of the population. Advances in genomics, proteomics, microbiomics, and bioinformatics are changing the face of health care, and dentistry is morphing as a result of this new knowledge and these technologies. Personalized or individualized medicine will allow more accurate and confirmatory diagnostics and better prediction of an individual's risk for certain conditions or diseases and help define optimal interventions and treatments. Tissue engineering, stem cell therapies, and designer protein and gene therapy are all becoming a reality and will help advance oral health care well beyond our current abilities and expectations. This text helps present our current diagnostic and therapeutic approaches for managing developmental defects of teeth and some craniofacial defects. This chapter provides a framework for our current understanding of the genetic and environmental etiologies associated with these conditions and directions for future diagnostics and therapies.

Introduction

Clinicians providing oral health care are challenged with myriad patients presenting with diverse developmental anomalies of the dental and craniofacial complex. While some of these anomalies are quite common and more easily diagnosed and may present the need for only minor deviations from traditional treatment approaches, others will present tremendous challenges in both their diagnosis and management. The number of conditions affecting development of the dentition are numerous and varied and are caused by both environmental and genetic etiologies. Extending this to the craniofacial complex further broadens the number of disorders, defects, and syndromes afflicting humans and their oral and craniofacial health. Developmental and hereditary disorders of the craniofacial and dental

J.T. Wright, DDS, MS
Department of Pediatric Dentistry,
James Bawden Distinguished Professor,
University of North Carolina School
of Dentistry, CB #7450, Brauer Hall 228,
Chapel Hill, NC 27599-7450, USA
e-mail: tim_wright@unc.edu

J.T. Wright (ed.), *Craniofacial and Dental Developmental Defects: Diagnosis and Management*,
DOI 10.1007/978-3-319-13057-6_1, © Springer International Publishing Switzerland 2015

complex vary in their prevalence, morbidity, and need for unique oral health-care management approaches. Providing optimal oral health care is predicated on having a basic understanding of the patient's underlying systemic and craniofacial condition, their current and future risk for developing oral pathology, and having the skills to diagnose their conditions and manage the patient's oral health needs. Depending on the condition and its complexity, this can involve a team of oral and medical health-care providers.

There are many online resources that can assist clinicians in their efforts to understand technologies related to genetics and current diagnostic approaches [28]. For example, there are numerous online primers to review basic genetics, how to obtain a family history and construct a pedigree, databases of hereditary conditions and teratogens, and many useful resources to evaluate the current knowledge and evidence for the diagnosis and treatment of craniofacial and dental conditions. While most schools of dentistry offer limited curricular time related to genomics and recent approaches to high-throughput genetic analysis, these new technologies are having an increasingly greater impact on health care [11, 13]. In this chapter we also provide directions and web addresses to some sites that are useful when seeking new knowledge on the etiologies and management of developmental defects of the craniofacial complex and teeth. One such example is the National Coalition for Health Professional Education in Genetics (NCHPEG – http://www.nchpeg.org/dentistry/index.php) that is transitioning to The Jackson Laboratories. This site provides information for dentists and hygienists to aid their understanding on the fundamentals of genetics and provide dentally relevant scenarios to help build skills in patient evaluation and family history taking. If you are confronted with a patient that has a clinical presentation that could be hereditary and they have not been diagnosed, a recommendation can be made for referral back to their primary care physician or to medical genetics. Information on specific genetic tests that are currently available, how to find a geneticist in your area, and other information can be found online at the National Institutes of Health site Genetics Home Reference (http://ghr.nlm.nih.gov/).

The goal of this chapter is to provide an overview of the diverse etiologies of craniofacial defects, our current knowledge of these etiologies, and how clinicians can access information related to a specific clinical diagnosis and its etiology. This information will provide a framework for the following chapters that provide greater detail on the diagnosis and management of conditions affecting the craniofacial complex and dentition.

Craniofacial Developmental Anomalies

The etiologies of dental and craniofacial defects are diverse and include environmental causes, genetics, and interactions between the two. As our knowledge expands regarding the causes and pathogenesis of developmental defects, it is incumbent on practitioners to stay current with diagnostic approaches and online resources that can provide valuable access to data and up-to-date information. There are thousands of hereditary conditions caused by changes in our genetic material. These conditions are caused by numerical or structural chromosomal changes, alteration in genes, and/or alteration of mitochondrial DNA. The frequency of chromosomal abnormalities is about 1–250 live births (March of Dimes – http://www.marchofdimes.com/; Center for Disease Control – http://www.cdc.gov/ncbddd/birthdefects/data.html) and 1 out of every 33 babies in the United States is born with a birth defect [5]. Some of the more common chromosomal abnormalities include Down syndrome (about 1–750 births involving chromosome 21), Klinefelter syndrome (1 in about 750 boys involving XXY), and Turner syndrome (1 in about 3,500 girls involving only one X chromosome). Table 1.1 shows the distribution of the nearly 8,000 hereditary conditions (Table 1.1) and their suspected or known mode of inheritance [21] . Virtually all of the chromosomal abnormalities and the majority of the Mendelian traits have associated craniofacial developmental anomalies. These developmental defects are diverse in their presentation with variants such as clefting, craniosynostosis, hemifacial microsomia, and vascular malformations being some of the more common craniofacial

Table 1.1 Conditions with Mendelian inheritance listed on OMIM June 2014

OMIM entry	Autosomal	X linked	Y linked	Mitochondrial	Totals
Phenotype described Molecular basis known	3,814	285	4	28	4,131
Phenotype described Molecular basis not known	1,562	134	5	0	1,701
Phenotypes with suspected Mendelian basis	1,738	115	2	0	1,855
	7,114	534	11	28	7,687

conditions. Because many of these disorders have other associated systemic and medical issues, it is important for the oral health-care provider to familiarize themselves with diverse manifestations that can accompany many developmental defects of the dentition and craniofacial complex. If a diagnosis is unknown or craniofacial anomalies are being identified and evaluated for the first time, a referral to the patient's physician or to medical genetics may be useful for further evaluation. For example, an individual with Down syndrome (OMIM #190685) is likely to have hypodontia (about 40 % of cases) and are at increased risk for developing periodontal disease. Additionally, they are likely to have an associated cardiac defect (about 40 % of cases) and have an increased risk for certain types of cancer like acute lymphocytic leukemia and thyroid dysfunction (about 20–50 %) [7]. Understanding a patient's dental and craniofacial condition and the potential for associated health risks is essential to providing the best health care. Associations between dental and craniofacial manifestations and systemic health are illustrated by many of the examples in this text.

In addition to hereditary etiologies, there are many environmental conditions associated with craniofacial malformations. There are numerous teratogens that can cause variable craniofacial phenotypes including ethanol, 13-cis retinoic acid (RA, Accutane), the antimetabolite methotrexate, periods of hypoxia, ionizing radiation, or hyperthermic stress [29]. The Center for Disease Control (CDC) and other groups have excellent information on teratogens that are associated with birth defects. The CDC reports that 50 % of pregnant women take four or more medications with

the number of women and medications taken during pregnancy increasing over the past several decades (http://www.cdc.gov/pregnancy/features/MedUsePregnancy-keyfindings.html) [19].

Birth defects are thus etiologically diverse and continue to be a major cause of developmental defects of the craniofacial and dental complex [22]. These different conditions present a plethora of clinical manifestations that often require the support of a diverse team of clinical health-care providers to address each individual's medical, psychosocial, and oral health-care needs. The greater the diversity of manifestations, the more likely it is that additional team members with unique expertise and knowledge will need to be involved. An example of this is the cleft lip/palate team (see Chap. 8) which will have diverse team membership to address the many different issues that accompany these conditions [32]. Whether individuals with developmental defects are cared for by a recognized team or by a community-based team of health-care providers, it is critical that effective interprofessional communication between these providers take place. Interprofessional communication will aid in obtaining a timely and accurate diagnosis and help optimize the efficiency and effectiveness of assisting the individual in the management of their health-care needs.

Developmental Defects Affecting the Dentition

Developmental defects can influence virtually every aspect of the dentition including the shape, color, size, number, composition, and the eruption

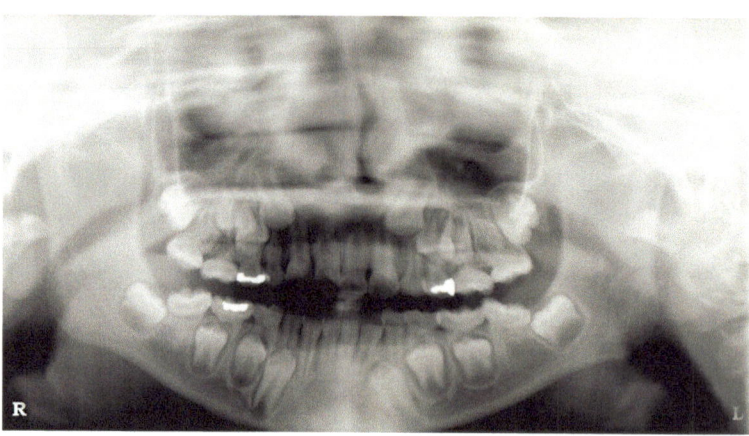

Fig. 1.1 The molar malformation that is referred to as molar incisor malformation is readily evident in this panoramic radiograph that shows the second primary and first permanent molars and maxillary permanent incisors are all affected

and exfoliation of teeth. The human dentition begins to develop at 6 weeks in utero as the oral epithelium invaginates to initiate tooth bud formation. The molecular controls that regulate the remarkable signaling and communication between the oral ectoderm and ectomesenchyme and subsequent processes related to cell differentiation, extracellular matrix formation, mineralization, and tooth eruption are extremely complex [2, 31]. It is likely that 10,000 or more genes are involved in the making of a human tooth. Depending on the specific tooth, it takes months to years to develop a single tooth and many years to develop the primary and then permanent dentition [16]. Given the complexity and long duration required for development of the dentitions, it is not surprising that there are many different environmental insults and genetic conditions that can result in a wide variety of dental defects and manifestations [25, 27].

The exact number of developmental defects is not known, but it certainly is in the hundreds with new conditions still being described in the literature. For example, a newly described condition that affects the first permanent molar and sometimes permanent incisors (molar incisor malformation – MIM) has just recently been described for the first time [15, 34]. The first permanent molars have a thin pulp chamber and abnormal root formation, and the etiology and prevalence are unknown at this time (Fig. 1.1). There are many known hereditary and environmental conditions associated with abnormalities in tooth number (both too many and too few). The medical history, in some cases, will readily provide the cause for missing teeth, such as

a child received extensive head and neck radiation and/or chemotherapy for cancer while the dentition was in its early developmental stages [8]. In other cases, the etiology will be more elusive as there may be a noncontributory medical history and no family history of missing teeth. As will be discussed in Chaps. 3 and 4, congenitally missing teeth can be associated with a syndromic condition, or it can occur as a nonsyndromic condition.

Teeth can form abnormally with defects in the compositions and/or structure of the enamel and/or dentin as discussed in Chaps. 6 and 7. These conditions can have significant psychosocial implications due to the importance of oral esthetics in our current society [6]. Their management often begins with eruption of the first primary tooth and continues throughout the life of the patient. Teeth may display normal crown formation but fail to erupt (Chap. 2) or may be lost prematurely (Chap. 3). Each of these different clinical manifestations provides critical diagnostic clues and will require different approaches in their management. Depending on the specific defects, a diverse dental team with expertise in a variety of areas could be needed to provide optimal oral health care over the life of the patients.

Accessing Information and Useful Databases

There are many resources that are readily available to clinicians that provide a plethora to wealth of information on conditions with craniofacial and genetic anomalies. The Internet has many different types of websites and available information. A number of very useful sites are sponsored by the National Center for Biotechnology Information (NCBI) which is a division of the National Library of Medicine. Established in 1988, NCBI creates automated systems for storing and analyzing knowledge about molecular biology, biochemistry, and genetics that can be used by researchers and health-care workers. One valuable NCBI site for clinicians is Online Mendelian Inheritance in Man (OMIM http://www.ncbi.nlm.nih.gov/omim/). This website catalogs hereditary conditions and provides information regarding clinical summaries of features, prognosis, genetic information, and direct links to references in PubMed. Each entry of a condition or gene is given a catalog number that can be used to help access the database. For example, Down syndrome is designated as OMIM # 190685. Clinicians can query this database to help access information on the clinical description of hereditary conditions and their etiology, if it is known. The OMIM database, while still incomplete, provides a wealth of information on hereditary conditions and is updated regularly. We have provided the OMIM numbers throughout this text to assist you in searching for additional information on conditions so you will be better able to diagnose and manage the oral health-care needs of your patients.

Family support groups often have extremely helpful information for both oral health-care providers and families. There are even family support groups for some of the very rare conditions. Many of these organizations have very informative websites that define the condition and have information on the current medical and dental management and information of the latest research being conducted on the diagnosis and treatment of the condition, for example, the National Foundation for Ectodermal Dysplasias, Osteogenesis Imperfecta Foundation, National Down Syndrome Society, and Cleft Palate Foundation to name just a few. Another excellent resource to get accurate information about rare conditions is the Office of Rare Disease Research sponsored by NIH (http://rarediseases.info.nih.gov/).

Taking a Family History

Taking a family medical history is often the critical first step in obtaining an accurate diagnosis and working with medical teams and making appropriate referrals [24]. The family medical history provides essential information for assessing whether a clinical condition may be associated with environmental causes and for assessing the potential mode of inheritance of developmental dental and craniofacial defects. Many medical organizations recommend evaluation of three generations and carefully assessing the presence of conditions in family members (e.g., American Society of Clinical Oncology, National Society of Genetic Counselors, American Medical Association). Knowledge of an individual's family medical history is the foundation for assessing the health and risk of disease for many different conditions ranging from cancer to dental caries. Constructing a pedigree is a useful way of systematically taking a family history and recording potentially affected family members. There are numerous online resources that provide tutorials on taking a family history and constructing informative pedigrees (http://www.geneticseducation. nhs.uk/mededu/identifying-those-at-risk/taking-a-genetic-family-history). Another tool that can be used to help take a family medical history can be found on the US Department of Health and Human Services website (http://www.hhs.gov/familyhistory/portrait/). Including a question on the health history that asks whether the patient has any familial or hereditary dental or health conditions is helpful in assessing each patient. Specific questions regarding a particular phenotype (e.g., missing teeth, enamel defects, etc.) can then be asked and detailed in the history and through construction of a pedigree.

As an example, one might ask the parent of a child who has exfoliated a tooth that has not been traumatized at age 18 months whether the child's siblings, biological parents, or biological grandparent had early loss of teeth. In this example, the parents respond that the child's older sister has no dental problems, but the father and paternal grandmother have a similar history of early tooth loss. The most useful way to display this family history

Fig. 1.2 Oral health-care providers should become versed in documenting family histories using the accepted convention of pedigree construction as illustrated in this example of a family having a trait that is transmitted as an autosomal dominant condition

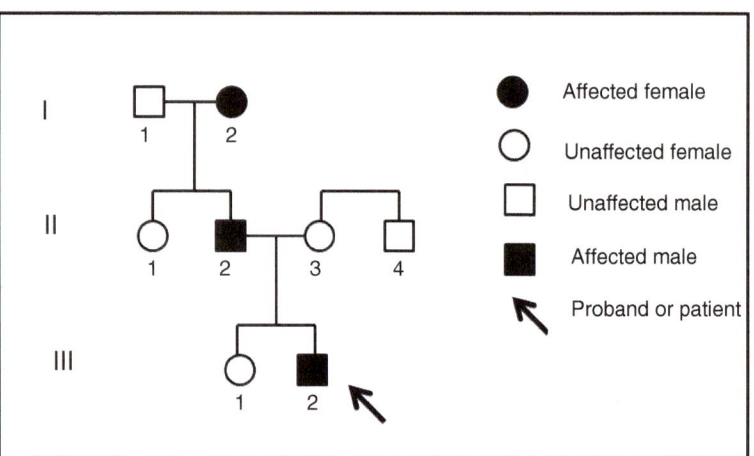

is in the form of a pedigree (Fig. 1.2). Pedigrees can be readily constructed with any computer program that can draw squares and circles. In this example, the pedigree does suggest there is a heritable risk for early tooth loss and that this trait can be transmitted from male to male and female to male suggesting an autosomal dominant mode of inheritance. This family medical history provides critical information for risk assessment and for helping direct further genetic studies that can help confirm the diagnosis.

Taking a family history provides invaluable information for risk assessment and diagnosis but also serves as a mechanism to build rapport with the family. Engaging the patient to elicit the family history will help educate them as to the cause and nature of the condition and to help them understand the prediction for possible diagnoses and prognosis for the condition. The hereditary conditions that affect the craniofacial and dental complex will be best managed when the patient's phenotype and the family history of the conditions consequences are considered in developing approaches in the management and or treatment of the problem.

Novel and Emerging Treatments and Therapeutic Approaches

There are incredible new approaches to manage and treat patients that address a broad range of developmental defects of the dental and craniofacial complex. Designer proteins to replace missing gene products, stem cell therapies, tissue engineering, gene therapy, and other biotechnologies are being extensively developed and are being incorporated into health care. For example, a variety of approaches are now being explored to rebuild the dental pulp [1]. One such approach involves seeding dental pulp stem cells in biodegradable scaffolds that are exposed to dentin-derived morphogenic factors. Under these conditions, the stem cells can give rise to a pulp-like tissue capable of generating new dentin [23].

Stem cell approaches also are being used to assist in the treatment of a wide array of craniofacial defects. Depending on the tissue and defect, there are many challenges to successful treatment. However, studies on the stem cells in periodontal regeneration and alveolar bone augmentation are showing good promise [3]. Autologous bone grafts and existing approaches have many limitations for managing large craniofacial skeletal defects. Innovative scaffold design, complemented by stem cell-based therapy and growth factor enhancement, is providing new approaches that will advance our ability to effectively manage developmental defects of the craniofacial complex [10, 30].

As our knowledge of genes and the proteins they code for builds, coupled with advancement in our ability to design and generate designer proteins, the potential for novel therapeutic approaches will multiple. One incredible example of this treatment approach is the development of a designer protein replacement for people with X-linked hypohidrotic ectodermal dysplasia (XHED). Males with XHED have sparse hair, decreased sweat ability to sweat, and hypodontia. The gene *EDA1* codes for the protein ectodysplasin, and mutations in this gene can cause XHED. A protein replacement has been developed and tested in mice and dogs that have mutations in their *EDA1* gene [4, 18]. Injections of the protein both pre- and postnatally are able to produce development of more normal dentitions [12]. This treatment approach is now being tested in phase II trials in humans. Other approaches to developing entire teeth from cell and tissue culture also are showing promise and being tested in animal models. To find out if there are clinical trials being conducted on a particular condition, you can search the Clinical Trials website that is a service of the NIH (http://www.clinicaltrials.gov/).

The advances that have been made in the development of new therapeutic approaches since publication of the human genome in 2003 have been remarkable. The powerful diagnostics that are now available will continue to advance our ability to determine an individual's genome and how it has been modified through epigenetic changes. Sequencing the first human genome was at an estimated cost of $3 billion, but now whole human genomes can be sequenced for a few thousand dollars. Not only has the cost lowered dramatically, but the time required to sequence a human genome also has been greatly reduced [17]. How this and other technological breakthroughs will change health care is not entirely clear although there is definitely a strong push in the direction of personalized health care. It is evident that health care will continue to evolve and that advances in diagnostics and novel therapeutic approaches will provide ever improving management of developmental defects of the dental and craniofacial complex.

Personalized Oral Health Care

During the last 150 or so years, medicine has moved into a scientifically based discipline with foundations in the germ theory, chemistry, biology, and pathology. In the 2000s, there has been a tremendous transformation due to advances in genomics, proteomics, microbiomics, metabolomics, and our ability to understand the fundamental mechanism of health and disease and to predict outcomes more effectively than ever (Fig. 1.3). Clinicians armed with information concerning their patients' conditions, their specific phenotypic features, and how the dental and/ or craniofacial tissues are affected will be equipped to assist them in having the best possible oral health. It is well known that every patient is different and that approaches to preventing, managing, and treating a patient with the goal to achieve optimal oral health is done at the individual level. Personalized health care in medicine has tremendous ramifications for many diseases known to have a genetic component to its etiology such as diabetes, cancer, and cardiovascular disease. Most of the advances using personalized health care have been in the diagnosis and treatment of cancer where knowing the tumor genotype or what genes are mutated can help elucidate what types of treatments are likely to be effective. Personalized oral health care is in its infancy with very few publications on the topic at this time [9, 14]. As more data is gathered on whole genomes from many different individuals and we understand the relationship between the genome and diverse states of health, and risk and disease, we will be better able to apply this information to improve diagnostics and treatment for our patients. Knowledge of the genetic contribution to the many conditions affecting the oral and craniofacial complex will allow an individual and practitioners to help better identify their patients' disease risk and diagnose hereditary conditions. It is thought that a large portion of the most common diseases affecting oral health have a significant genetic component, and there has been research on genes that are associated with dental caries and periodontal disease [20, 26, 33]. Dental caries (about 50 % of risk is genetic) and periodontal disease (about 35 % risk is genetic) are both complex diseases that result from environmental conditions that interact with the host who has a genetically defined risk and resistance to the disease. This also is true for dental maloc-

Fig. 1.3 Information from numerous sources will allow the integration of information from different factors or domains that influence health and disease risk allowing a personalized approach to managing oral health

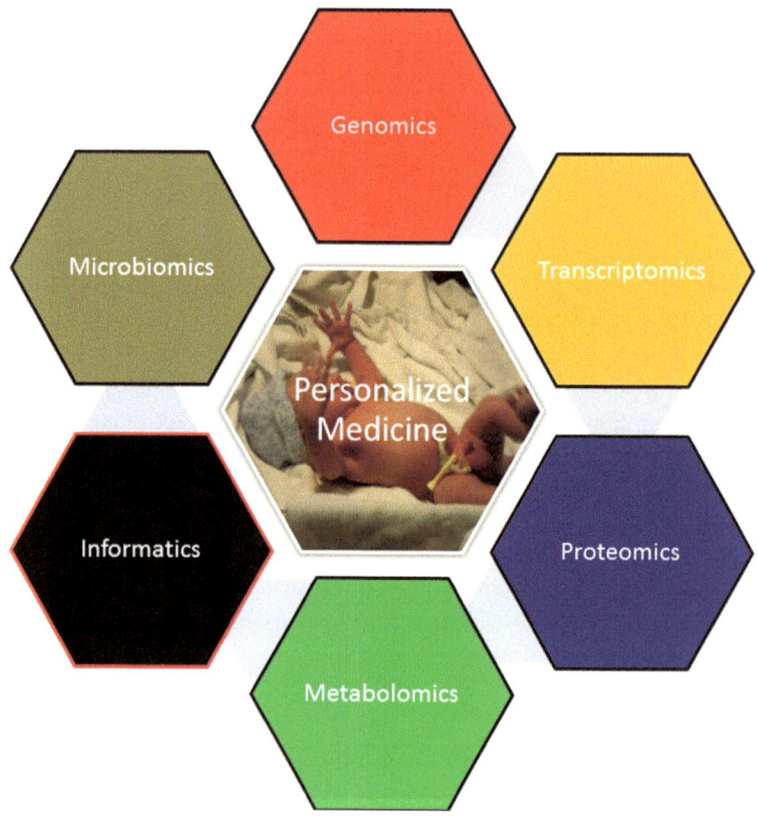

clusions with investigators stating that 50 % or more of malocclusions are associated with genetics [35]. Managing conditions that have significant genetic determinants in their etiology and or progression could be markedly improved by harnessing the knowledge of the individual's inherent risk and resistance. Interventions could be targeted more specifically, and the timing and duration of treatment could be more objectively predicted and applied. This is illustrated in Chap. 6 on tooth eruption where a diagnosis of primary failure of tooth eruption caused by a *PTH1R* gene mutation is not treatable using typical orthodontic tooth movement. Having the diagnosis determines the prognosis and helps direct what successful treatments might be applied. As our knowledge of the human genome and its function continues to advance, our ability to use this information to improve and individualize oral health care will progress.

Conclusion

We live in an age of rapid scientific and medical advancement, and clinicians are challenged to keep up with the ever-growing body of knowledge related to the diagnosis and management of the dentition and craniofacial complex. As we move forward into an era of new diagnostics and therapeutics fueled by projects such as the human genome, microbiome, and pharmacogenetics, oral health-care providers will be called upon to integrate information from these new fields of knowledge into personalized health care for their patients. This text is meant to provide you useful information on the diagnosis and management of some of the more common conditions that oral health-care providers may encounter. More importantly, it is meant to provide a framework and guidance as to how and where additional information can be obtained for the many conditions not covered in this text.

References

1. Albuquerque MT, Valera MC, Nakashima M, Nor JE, Bottino MC. Tissue-engineering-based strategies for regenerative endodontics. J Dent Res. 2014;93(12):1222–31.

2. Biggs LC, Mikkola ML. Early inductive events in ectodermal appendage morphogenesis. Semin Cell Dev Biol. 2014;25–26:11–21.

3. Bright R, Hynes K, Gronthos S, Bartold PM. Periodontal ligament-derived cells for periodontal regeneration in animal models: a systematic review. J Periodont Res. 2014. doi:10.1111/jre.12205. [Epub ahead of print]

4. Casal ML, Lewis JR, Mauldin EA, Tardivel A, Ingold K, Favre M, et al. Significant correction of disease after postnatal administration of recombinant ectodysplasin A in canine X-linked ectodermal dysplasia. Am J Hum Genet. 2007;81(5):1050–6.

5. CDC CfDCaP. Update on overall prevalence of major birth defects Atlanta, Georgia, 1978–2005. MMWR Morb Mortal Wkly Rep. 2008;57(1):1–5.

6. Coffield KD, Phillips C, Brady M, Roberts MW, Strauss RP, Wright JT. The psychosocial impact of developmental dental defects in people with hereditary amelogenesis imperfecta. JADA. 2005;136(5):620–30.

7. Delabar JM, Theophile D, Rahmani Z, Chettouh Z, Blouin JL, Prieur M, et al. Molecular mapping of twenty-four features of Down syndrome on chromosome 21. Eur J Hum Genet. 1993;1(2):114–24.

8. Effinger KE, Migliorati CA, Hudson MM, McMullen KP, Kaste SC, Ruble K, et al. Oral and dental late effects in survivors of childhood cancer: a Children's Oncology Group report. Support Care Cancer. 2014;22(7):2009–19.

9. Giannobile WV, Kornman KS, Williams RC. Personalized medicine enters dentistry: what might this mean for clinical practice? J Am Dent Assoc. 2013;144(8):874–6.

10. Grimm WD, Dannan A, Giesenhagen B, Schau I, Varga G, Vukovic MA, et al. Translational research: palatal-derived ecto-mesenchymal stem cells from human palate: a new hope for alveolar bone and cranio-facial bone reconstruction. Int J Stem Cells. 2014;7(1):23–9.

11. Hart TC, Marrazita M, Wright JT. Molecular genetics and the paradigm shift in oral health care. Crit Rev Oral Biol. 2000;11:26–56.

12. Hermes K, Schneider P, Krieg P, Dang A, Huttner K, Schneider H. Prenatal therapy in developmental disorders: drug targeting via intra-amniotic injection to treat X-linked hypohidrotic ectodermal dysplasia. J Invest Dermatol. 2014;134:2985–7.

13. Johnson L, Genco RJ, Damsky C, Haden NK, Hart S, Hart TC, et al. Genetics and its implications for clinical dental practice and education: report of panel 3 of the Macy study. J Dent Educ. 2008;72(2):86–94.

14. Kornman KS, Duff GW. Personalized medicine: will dentistry ride the wave or watch from the beach? J Dent Res. 2012;91(7):8S–11.

15. Lee HS, Kim SH, Kim SO, Lee JH, Choi HJ, Jung HS, et al. A new type of dental anomaly: molar-incisor malformation (MIM). Oral Surg Oral Med Oral Pathol Oral Radiol. 2014;118(1):101–9.e103.

16. Lunt RC, Law DB. A review of the chronology of calcification of deciduous teeth. J Am Dent Assoc. 1974;89:872–9.

17. Mardis ER. A decade's perspective on DNA sequencing technology. Nature. 2011;470(7333):198–203.

18. Mauldin EA, Gaide O, Schneider P, Casal ML. Neonatal treatment with recombinant ectodysplasin prevents respiratory disease in dogs with X-linked ectodermal dysplasia. Am J Med Genet A. 2009;149A(9):2045–9.

19. Mitchell AA, Gilboa SM, Werler MM, Kelley KE, Louik C, Hernandez-Diaz S, et al. Medication use during pregnancy, with particular focus on prescription drugs: 1976–2008. Am J Obstet Gynecol. 2011;205(1):51.e51–8.

20. Mucci LA, Bjorkman L, Douglass CW, Pedersen NL. Environmental and heritable factors in the etiology of oral diseases – a population-based study of Swedish twins. J Dent Res. 2005;84(9):800–5.

21. Online Mendelian Inheritance in Man. WWW URL: http://www3.ncbi.nlm.gov/omim/ version. Baltimore: Center for Medical Genetics, Johns Hopkins University and National Center for Biotechnology Information, National Library of Medicine; 2014.

22. Parker SE, Mai CT, Canfield MA, Rickard R, Wang Y, Meyer RE, et al. Updated national birth prevalence estimates for selected birth defects in the United States, 2004–2006. Birth defects research Part A. Clin Mol Teratol. 2010;88(12):1008–16.

23. Piva E, Silva AF, Nor JE. Functionalized scaffolds to control dental pulp stem cell fate. J Endod. 2014;40(4):S33–40.

24. Rich EC, Burke W, Heaton CJ, Haga S, Pinsky L, Short MP, et al. Reconsidering the family history in primary care. J Gen Intern Med. 2004;19(3):273–80.

25. Seow WK. Developmental defects of enamel and dentine: challenges for basic science research and clinical management. Aust Dent J. 2014;59(S1):51–4.

26. Slayton R. Genetics may have a significant contribution to dental caries while microbial acid production appears to be modulated by the environment. J Evid Based Dent Pract. 2006;6(2):185–6.

27. Small B, Murray J. Enamel opacities: prevalence, classification and aetiological considerations. J Dent. 1978;6(1):33–42.

28. Stark LA, Pompei K. Winner of science prize for online resources in education. Making genetics easy to understand. Science. 2010;327(5965):538–9.

29. Sulik KK, Cook CS, Webster WS. Teratogens and craniofacial malformations: relationships to cell death. Development. 1988;103 Suppl:213–31.

30. Tevlin R, McArdle A, Atashroo D, Walmsley GG, Senarath-Yapa K, Zielins ER, et al. Biomaterials for craniofacial bone engineering. J Dent Res. 2014;93(12):1187–95.

31. Thesleff I. Epithelial-mesenchymal signalling regulating tooth morphogenesis. J Cell Sci. 2003;116(Pt 9): 1647–8.

32. Vargervik K, Oberoi S, Hoffman WY. Team care for the patient with cleft: UCSF protocols and outcomes. J Craniofac Surg. 2009;20(2):1668–71.

33. Vieira AR, Modesto A, Marazita ML. Caries: review of human genetics research. Caries Res. 2014;48(5): 491–506.

34. Witt CV, Hirt T, Rutz G, Luder HU. Root malformation associated with a cervical mineralized diaphragm – a distinct form of tooth abnormality? Oral Surg Oral Med Oral Pathol Oral Radiol. 2014; 117(4):e311–9.

35. Zanardi GPW, Frazier-Bowers SA. The future of dentistry: how will personalized medicine affect orthodontic treatment? Dental Press J Orthod. 2012;17: 3–6.

Failure of Tooth Eruption: Diagnosis and Management

Sylvia A. Frazier-Bowers and Heather M. Hendricks

Abstract

Tooth eruption disorders are diverse in their etiologies and can be difficult to diagnose. Management of tooth eruption disorders is predicated largely on establishing a correct diagnosis and will depend on the clinical phenotype (e.g., what teeth are affected, severity of the condition, patient age, and health status). The etiologies of abnormalities in tooth eruption include inadequate space, presence of obstructions such as cysts, ankyloses, and hereditary conditions, to name just a few. Treatment approaches will depend on the age of the patient, number of teeth involved, diagnosis, treatment cost, and other factors. The goal of this chapter is to provide a foundation for the diagnosis of tooth eruption disorders and review some of the available treatment options.

Introduction

The clinical management of tooth eruption disorders presents a significant challenge, largely because the diagnosis is so complex and the primary mechanism of eruption itself is poorly understood. The etiologies of tooth eruption disorders are diverse and include environmental stresses

S.A. Frazier-Bowers, DDS, PhD (✉)
Associate Professor, 7450 Brauer Hall,
Department of Orthodontics,
Chapel Hill, NC, 27599, (919) 537-3758
e-mail: sylvia_frazier-bowers@unc.edu

H.M. Hendricks DDS
Department of Orthodontics, University of North
Carolina at Chapel Hill,
Chapel Hill, NC, USA
e-mail: jan.lewerenz@googlemail.com

such as trauma and a variety of genetic conditions such as primary failure of eruption (PFE, OMIM #125350) and cleidocranial dysplasia (OMIM #119600). A search for tooth and eruption on OMIM reveals 119 conditions listed as having tooth eruption issues that range from natal teeth (OMIM #187050) to various forms of amelogenesis imperfecta (OMIM #s130900, 204690, 613211). Individuals with different forms of osteogenesis imperfecta (see Chap. 7) are at increased risk for developing dentigerous cysts around developing teeth that can obstruct normal tooth eruption. Gingival overgrowth, such as occurs in a variety of conditions (e.g., gingival fibromatosis with hypertrichosis, OMIM #135400), has disturbed tooth eruption. It is helpful to begin with a clear understanding of what is known about tooth eruption, including normal and abnormal events,

J.T. Wright (ed.), *Craniofacial and Dental Developmental Defects: Diagnosis and Management*,
DOI 10.1007/978-3-319-13057-6_2, © Springer International Publishing Switzerland 2015

to provide the necessary foundation to diagnose and manage eruption disorders. The diversity of these conditions and their etiologies make the diagnosis and subsequent treatment difficult.

In the permanent human dentition, the normal process of eruption can be divided into major clinical stages – preemergent and postemergent. The preemergent eruption stage is the most important in the initiation of the eruption process; combined resorption and eruption process facilitates eruption of the permanent tooth [1]. Resorption of alveolar bone and primary tooth roots overlying the crown of the erupting permanent tooth facilitates the resultant eruption of the permanent tooth; this coordinated process moves the tooth into the pathway cleared by resorption. It is the uncoupling of these two processes, eruption and resorption, in naturally occurring human conditions (i.e., primary failure of eruption or osteopetrosis) that illustrates that the two processes are actually separate. For instance, in osteopetrosis (OMIM #259700), a syndromic condition, teeth fail to erupt due to the absence of an eruptive pathway resulting from a defective metabolic process of the bone [2]. In this case the resorption process is faulty. In PFE, a nonsyndromic disorder, the opposite scenario exists; the resorptive pathway is cleared, but the tooth fails to erupt [3, 4]. Postemergent tooth eruption disorders also occur. Ankylosis is a relatively prevalent condition in the primary dentition (prevalence: about 7–8 % of children have one or more affected teeth) and results from a loss of normal periodontal ligament and the bone attaching directly to the tooth root. Ankylosis occurs more commonly in the siblings of children that have ankyloses, is more common in the mandibular dentition, and more commonly affects teeth that do not have a permanent successor (often a primary molar with no secondary dentition premolar) [39]. Ankylosed primary teeth also are commonly associated with other dental anomalies in a high percentage of cases including tooth agenesis, microdont lateral incisors, and palatally displaced permanent canine teeth [40].

It is useful to begin our exploration of eruption anomalies by contrasting the molecular events surrounding eruption and, by extension, these two diametrically opposed scenarios. Molecular studies have revealed that eruption is, in fact, a tightly coordinated process, regulated by a series of signaling events between the dental follicle and the alveolar bone [5]. As indicated above, in osteopetrosis, the resorptive process is faulty due to an osteoclast defect. This is in contrast to a complete failure of the primary eruption mechanism that is not associated with defective osteoclasts [3, 7]. In PFE, a genetic alteration in the parathyroid hormone receptor 1 (*PTH1R*) gene [4, 8] further confirms the molecular basis of tooth eruption; a mutation in the *PTH1R* gene results in a striking failure of eruption that is hereditary. This finding is significant as nonsyndromic eruption disturbances are difficult to distinguish from one another (i.e., ankylosis versus PFE or a mechanical obstruction of eruption) [6]. This finding is significant as nonsyndromic eruption disturbances are difficult to distinguish from one another (i.e., ankylosis versus delayed eruption) [6].

Theories Associated with Preemergent Tooth Eruption

The normal eruption of permanent teeth is highly varied and multifactorial. In order to properly categorize eruption disorders, it is critical to have a thorough understanding of normal eruption. Previous studies using implants and cephalometric radiography have shown that as the developing tooth bud forms, it remains in the same location in the bone [9], and it is from this point that eruption begins. The stages of eruption are determined by whether or not the tooth has emerged into the oral cavity.

While preemergent tooth eruption is defined by the initial eruptive movements that occur at the beginning of root formation and alveolar bone resorption in the eruption pathway, postemergent eruption is marked by the relatively rapid eruption after the tooth has entered the oral cavity. In preemergent eruption, the developing

Fig. 2.1 (**a**) Type I primary failure of eruption in a developing dentition (7.5-year-old child). The right posterior segment shows a progressive eruption failure in the upper and lower arches with an eruption pathway that is clear. The left posterior segment does not appear affected. (**b**) Failure of eruption due to a bony pathway that is not clear. The alveolar bone can still be observed coronal to the erupting first molar in the lower left quadrant. This scenario often represents an idiopathic eruption failure due to some other pathology (i.e., not PFE or syndromic cause)

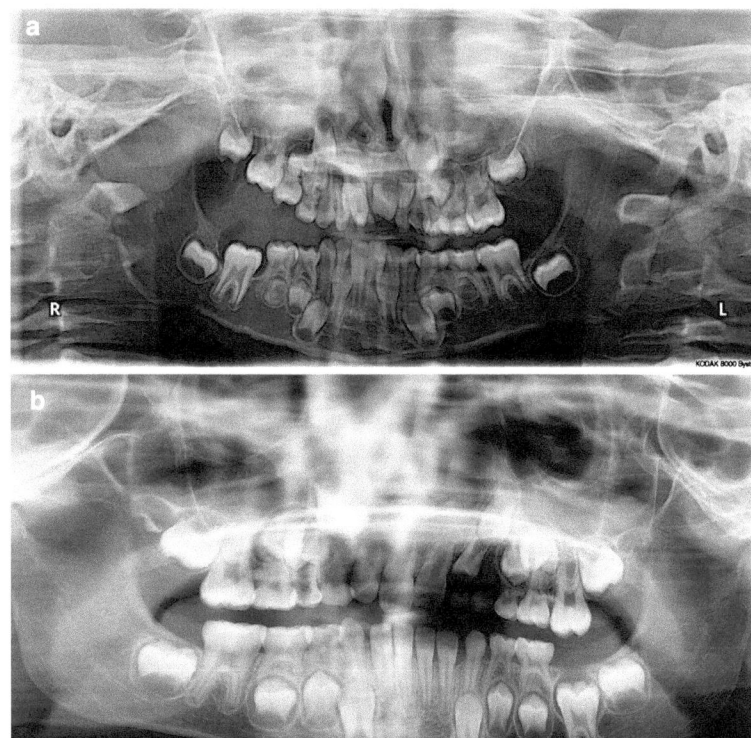

tooth moves occlusal and away from the point where root development is occurring. The precise mechanism of preemergent tooth eruption remains widely debated, but historical studies offer many lines of evidence for various theories [10–14]. Canonical theories in the recent literature include the "bone remodeling theory," the "hydrostatic theory," and the "follicle theory," which we will consider in detail below. Other historical theories that have been proposed include the "fibroblastic contraction theory" and those theories involving collagen maturation, localized variations in blood pressure or flow, alterations in the extracellular ground substances of the periodontal ligament, and the "root elongation theory." Briefly, the "fibroblastic contraction theory" hypothesizes that contraction of the fibroblast is responsible for the occlusal eruption of a tooth. Evidence in favor of this theory is the observation that fibroblasts move incisally along the erupting tooth [15] and that the contraction of fibroblasts generates significant force [16] to bring about eruption of the tooth. However, experiments in a rat model using lathyrogens (amino acid deriva-

tives that cause defective fibril formation when applied to the PDL) to weaken the periodontal ligaments did not show a significantly different rate of eruption when compared to untreated rats [17]. The lack of PDL organization in the unerupted tooth does not support the eruptive theory of preemergent collagen maturation.

In the "root formation theory" [18, 19], it is hypothesized that lengthening of the root causes pressure on the apical portion of the alveolar bone leading to obvious propulsion of the tooth into the oral cavity. This theory suggests that the pressure of a developing tooth root on the underlying bone causes osteogenesis apically and bone resorption coronal to the erupting tooth. This argument is weakened by the fact the teeth with root apices surgically removed erupt normally [20] and that when eruption of a tooth is prevented by surgically ligating a premolar tooth bud to the lower border of the mandible in a dog model, the eruption path was still cleared [12]. The human equivalent of this phenomenon can be observed in accidental ligation of a developing permanent tooth to the adjacent mandibular bone in the case of mandibular fractures *or* cases of PFE (Fig. 2.1a) where it is obvious that an eruption pathway has cleared but the tooth has failed to erupt to the occlusal plane. This is in direct contrast to a scenario where the eruption pathway is not cleared and eruption is essentially mechanically obstructed (Fig. 2.1b).

The remaining theories possibly offer the strongest explanation of tooth eruption, particularly in light of recent molecular biological advances [4, 5, 8]. However, these theories have fueled a debate of whether the bone "pushes" the teeth or the tooth "pulls" the bone with it during the eruption process. The "bone remodeling theory," originally proposed by Ten Cate [11] and endorsed by Wise et al. [14, 21], asserts that bone growth within the area apical to the developing tooth "pushes" the tooth during the eruption process. The consideration is whether this bone growth is causal and indeed represents the "motive force" described by Wise [14] or whether the bone growth occurs as a response to the occlusal movement of the developing tooth. Significant evidence exists in animal models to support this theory; experiments in rats reveal that the amount and duration of bone growth occurring at the apical base of the tooth is necessary and sufficient to propel the tooth into the oral cavity [14]. However, the fact remains that tooth eruption in humans occurs over a protracted time period with limited accessibility for study and the above studies in rodents may not parallel the human response; hence the complete understanding of events leading to eruption in humans remains elusive. The theory of preemergent eruption that most closely fits this model is the "dental follicle theory," which relates to the physiologic coupling of the resorptive eruption path formation and root development processes and contends that the dental follicle is necessary for eruption [12, 13]. This provides the most compelling explanation of the mechanism underlying tooth eruption. Moreover, it is this theory that aligns best with the "bone remodeling theory" and the association of the *PTH1R* gene with PFE. The follicle theory stems from classical studies in dogs where removal of the dental follicle prevented eruption [12, 13]. The dental follicle has since been shown to provide the environment and chemoattractants for monocytes

to differentiate into osteoclasts [5]; this facilitates the bone resorption necessary for normal tooth eruption. Specifically, stellate reticulum cells found in the dental follicle are observed to secrete parathyroid hormone-related peptide (PTHrP), which induces overexpression of colony-stimulating factor-1 (CSF1) and receptor activator of NF-kappaB ligand (RANKL) responsible for osteoclastogenesis [24, 25]. A concomitant overexpression of BMP2 that leads to osteogenesis is occurring in the apical end of the dental follicle [24] in a chronological and spatial fashion [21].

The complete explanation of the physiologic coupling of the eruption and resorption processes associated with preemergent tooth eruption is not yet fully understood, but we know that the molecular crosstalk surrounding the erupting tooth is somehow activated upon completion of the crown. We can therefore postulate that the rate-limiting factor of preemergent eruption is the resorptive pathway formed by osteoclast cells. Accordingly, a tooth embedded in the bone has the potential to begin to erupt after root formation is completed, as long as the eruptive pathway is mechanically cleared at the appropriate developmental stage. This natural phenomenon of a "clear pathway" forms the basis of the diagnostic rubric for eruption disorders discussed in detail below.

Theories Associated with Postemergent Tooth Eruption

Although the dominant theories of tooth eruption appear to correlate with the preemergent stage, the postemergent stage of eruption is central to some theories. Postemergent tooth eruption is defined as the eruption stage of a developing tooth after it has broken through the gingiva into the oral cavity. This stage continues until the tooth reaches the level of the occlusal plane and is in complete function and the overall growth of the jaws has completed. Postemergent eruption is further broken into four phases, the pre-functional spurt (rapid phase), the juvenile occlusal equilibrium (slower phase), the pubertal or adolescent eruptive spurt, and the adult occlusal equilibrium. After the gingival barrier is broken, the postemergent spurt results in rapid eruption until the tooth reaches the level of functional occlusion. As the tooth continues to erupt during its postemergent stage, the theory of "collagen cross-linking, contraction, and maturation" introduced above becomes more viable, due to the fact that the PDL indeed becomes more organized after the tooth comes into functional occlusion. This theory contends that increased organization in collagen cross-linking creates a propulsive thrust to facilitate eruption. Even though the tooth is subjected to occlusal forces, the actual eruption rate is increased.

The "hydrostatic pressure theory" occurs during postemergent eruption and is based on the ability of the extracellular matrix apical to the developing tooth to swell considerably (30–50 %) facilitating occlusal migration of the tooth [22, 23]. This theory asserts that increases in the periapical tissue fluid pressure (especially vasculature) push the tooth occlusally [11]. Moreover, human studies of premolar eruption following a local injection of vasodilators resulted in tooth eruption [23]. The argument against this theory is that a short-lived exposure to pharmacologic agents such as vasodilators would not be sufficient to sustain the long-term physiologic activity necessary for tooth eruption [14].

Postemergent Eruption and the Equilibrium Theory

After the functional plane is reached by the tooth, it undergoes the juvenile occlusal equilibrium, in which the eruption of the tooth is balanced in response to the vertical growth of the mandibular ramus. As the mandible grows vertically away from the maxilla, the teeth have more room to erupt occlusally in order to maintain occlusal contact with the opposing arch. This model of tooth eruption reinforces the idea that postemergent tooth eruption, after reaching functional occlusion, is controlled by forces impeding eruption, as opposed to encouraging forces. These balancing forces of masticatory function and the soft tissue pressures from the lips, cheeks, and tongue are the rate-limiting factors of postfunctional occlusal eruption [1]. However, studies have shown that lasting eruptive movement occurs while the teeth are not in contact, which supports the idea that most of the eruptive control is based on the light and continuous force of the soft tissues. While the mechanism itself is not fully understood, when this process of vertical growth and occlusal tooth eruption is not adequately matched, eruption problems arise, as seen with issues of ankylosis and other eruption disorders which can result in areas of posterior open bites and over-closed jaw relationships.

The last phase of postemergent eruption is called the adult occlusal equilibrium. In this continuous phase, teeth will continue to erupt at an extremely slow rate throughout adult life. It has been demonstrated that if a tooth is lost at any age, the opposing tooth has the ability to erupt more rapidly, demonstrating that the eruption mechanism remains active throughout life and is capable of producing significant tooth during any stage in the life cycle. Finally, both pre- and postemergent eruption stages play a significant role in clinical eruption disorders and form the basis of our diagnostic approach reviewed below.

Diagnosis of Tooth Eruption Problems

While rodent models and molecular advances lend some support to the various theories of eruption, the details of the entire process of tooth eruption, including the micro- and macro-environment, remain poorly understood. Nonetheless, the biological facts surrounding the proposed theories provide the basis for understanding and diagnosing clinical disorders of eruption. Accordingly, adopting a diagnostic system that uses biologically rather than clinically based categories would provide a more effective means of accurately distinguishing eruption disorders [26]. Such categories should include those based on (1) a biological dysfunction such as PFE or eruption failure secondary to a genetic syndrome [16] and/or (2) a physical obstruction such as mechanical failure, cysts, and lateral tongue pressure, for instance. Impacted teeth may potentially belong to either of the above categories depending upon the location of the impacted tooth (i.e., palatal canine impaction versus buccal canine impaction). While the occurrence of palatally impacted canines is hypothesized to be both multifactorial and genetic in origin [27–29], teeth can also become impacted secondary to an obstruction of the eruption pathway, such as crowded dental arches.

It is for this reason that a diagnostic rubric to distinguish eruption disorders must ask the necessary question "is the eruptive pathway clear?"

[30]. The answer to this creates the foundation for determining whether the eruption failure is due to an obstruction or not. The diagnostic rubric shown in Fig. 2.2a is based on studies that examined characteristics of eruption disorders; the accompanying case study (Fig. 2.2b, c) nicely illustrates how this tool can be utilized for a clinical diagnosis. The combination of objective

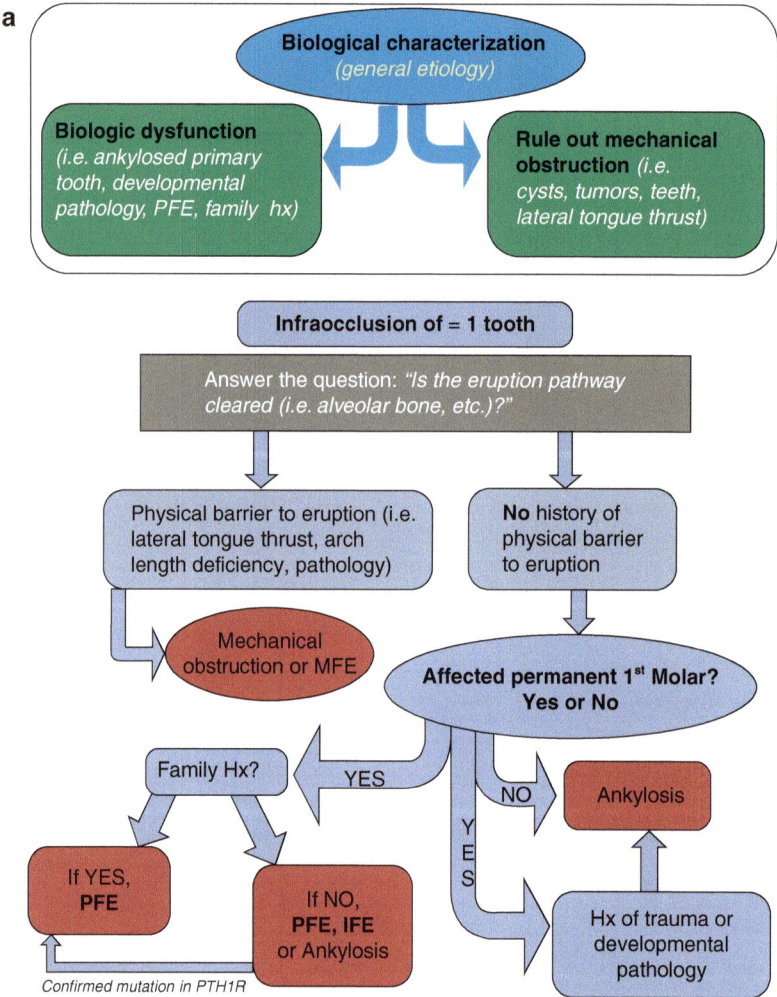

Fig. 2.2 (**a**) Diagnostic rubric for nonsyndromic eruption disorders based on a retrospective study of PFE subjects who carry a mutation in the *PTH1R* gene and those who do not. The flowchart provides a decision tree to allow a more systematic diagnosis of eruption disorders. Although there is still some uncertainty, initially sorting based on biological versus mechanical factors provides a sound basis to triage clinical scenarios (**b, c**). In the clinical scenario shown here, the natural history of this patient was extremely important. A differential diagnosis of the initial panoramic radiograph taken at the information gathering visit could be PFE or MFE. It was evident after acquiring historical radiographs (3 years earlier) that the cause of the eruption failure was an odontoma that was not removed before the 6 year molar was ready to erupt. Shown encircled is the unerupted 6 year molar in the 8 year old patient radiograph (2.2c) and the same molar at 11 years old that is now permanently impacted. Removal of the adjacent second premolar allowed eruption of the impacted molar and correction of the subsequent malocclusion. Reprinted from American Journal of Orthodontics and Dentofacial Orthopedics. Aug 144 (2)194–202

Fig. 2.2 (continued)

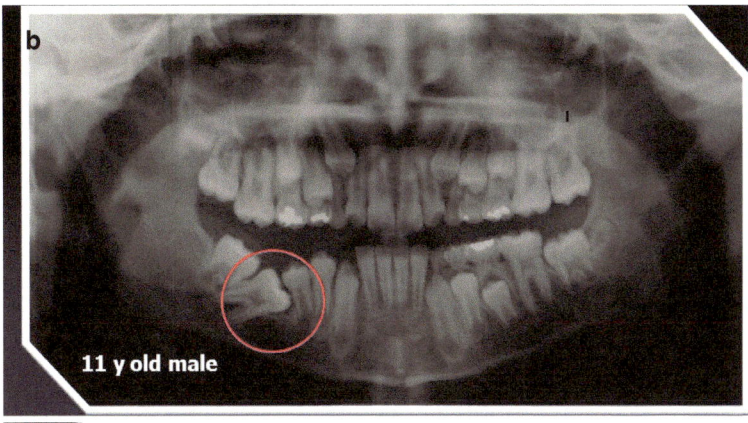

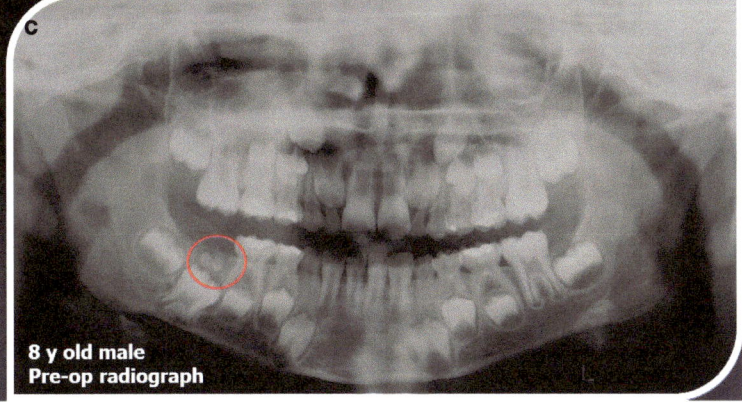

genetic information and clinical data from affected persons can be used to establish a genotype-phenotype correlation for PFE and, by extension, an objective diagnosis, i.e., determined by associating clinical (phenotypic) features with genetic (genotypic) analysis. Eruption disorders from a cohort of 64 patients were analyzed phenotypically and genetically in order to categorize them into clinical groups: (1) those definitively diagnosed with PFE through genetic analysis, (2) those that showed a mutation in *PTH1R* ($n = 11$; genetic PFE cohort), (3) patients diagnosed with PFE based on clinical records alone ($n = 47$; clinical PFE cohort), and (4) patients diagnosed with ankylosis based on clinical criteria ($N = 6$; clinical ankylosis cohort). Those in the ankylosis cohort had a confirmed history of trauma or were treated with extraction of the affected tooth or teeth and had successful orthodontic treatment of the remaining teeth. All other subjects were diagnosed with PFE based on history of unsuccessful orthodontic treatment or genetic analysis. For those PFE patients who underwent genetic (mutational) analysis, a mutation or polymorphism in the *PTH1R* gene was identified in 11 patients, and an unclassified nonfunctional single nucleotide polymorphism in *PTH1R* was identified in the remaining [30]. Based on the findings of the above study, collectively all PFE subjects (genetic cohort) had at least one affected first permanent molar; the affected teeth in each dental quadrant were adjacent to one another and had a supracrestal presentation (i.e., completely cleared eruption pathway, with no alveolar bone occlusal to the affected tooth). These criteria represent the hallmark features of PFE versus a mechanical obstruction since it is based on cases of PFE genetic cohort that were categorized based on objective genetic confirmation. Other classifications of PFE include type I versus type II PFE [7, 26]. Type I is marked by a progressive open bite from the anterior to the posterior of the dental arches, while type II presents similarly but with greater although inadequate eruption of a second molar (Fig. 2.3). In either case, we speculate that

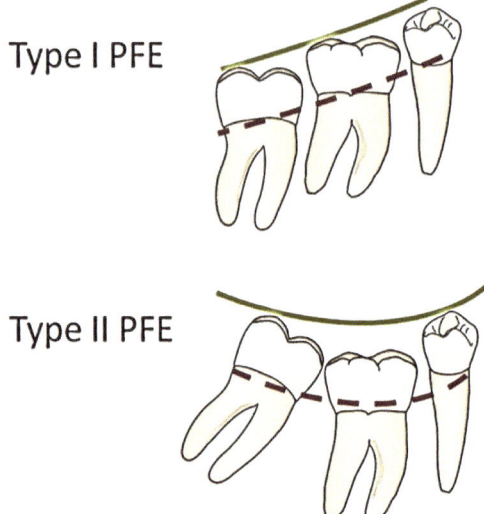

Type I PFE

Type II PFE

Fig. 2.3 Graphic representation of primary failure of eruption in type I and type II showing the progressive worsening of the posterior lateral open bite, to a lesser extent in type II PFE. Ankylosis occurs at about a 6.6% prevalence with mandibular primary molars more commonly affected than maxillary primary molars [38].

the eruption defect, which we now know is genetically controlled, is expressed at the same developmental time for all affected teeth but the predominant "molar" phenotype that we observe may be the result of a coordinated series of molecular events that act in a *temporally* and *spatially* specific manner such that posterior rather than anterior alveolar bone is affected. The exact reason for the variation in eruption potential between the first and second molars in type II is unknown but may be related to this same temporal and spatial specificity of expression.

Despite the more definitive criteria established through the eruption disorder rubric, difficulty still exists for those clinical situations that present with isolated ankylosis since it may initially appear indistinguishable from PFE. Ankylosis, or the fusion of a tooth to the bone in the absence of a periodontal ligament, can be thought of as a mechanical eruption failure, primarily because it can occur secondary to trauma and the fusion to the bone provides a mechanical barrier to eruption [31]. It is true that ankylosis can also occur secondarily from orthodontic forces applied to a tooth with a defective eruption mechanism as in

PFE [3]. The diagnosis of ankylosis can at times be made radiographically by the absence of a periodontal ligament space [32] and based on the absence of physiologic mobility and the sharp solid sound on percussion of the tooth [31]. However, the determination of an absent periodontal ligament space can be often misinterpreted on a radiograph (e.g., if ankylosis occurs in facial/lingual root surfaces, the PDL loss will not be visible on a 2D radiograph), making the diagnosis of ankylosis somewhat subjective [33]. In these instances, ankylosis can be difficult to distinguish from PFE. This fact has been exemplified in two siblings previously diagnosed with ankylosis that were re-diagnosed as PFE following identification of a mutation in the *PTH1R* gene [4] (Figs. 2.4a and 2.5). The two siblings diagnosed with ankylosis, later determined to be PFE, also have an affected mother (not shown) and brother (Fig. 2.6a–c) who harbor a mutation in *PTH1R*. In both cases treatment with a continuous archwire failed to correct the posterior open bite (Fig. 2.4c). It is therefore quite reasonable that many other cases previously diagnosed as ankylosis are in fact PFE since the clinical presentation of PFE due to a genetic defect shows great clinical variation and is similar to ankylosis [4, 8]. Hence, the recent identification of a gene associated with PFE not only contributes to our understanding of the specific biological mechanism underlying the eruption process, but it provides greater clarity to the various terminologies used to describe eruption failure.

In some clinical situations however, the diagnosis of ankylosis is rather straightforward and not confused with eruption failure – specifically, ankylosis associated with retained deciduous teeth. Despite the apparent distinction between ankylosis and PFE, the actual biologic differences remain elusive; ankylosis is indeed similar to PFE in that a familial tendency has been reported and an overall prevalence of 8.9%. This percentage increases with age in children [39]. As discussed earlier, ankylosis of primary molars occurs most frequently with agenesis of second premolars, which are the most common congenitally missing teeth second only to third molars [33, 34]. It is not uncommon to see that resorp-

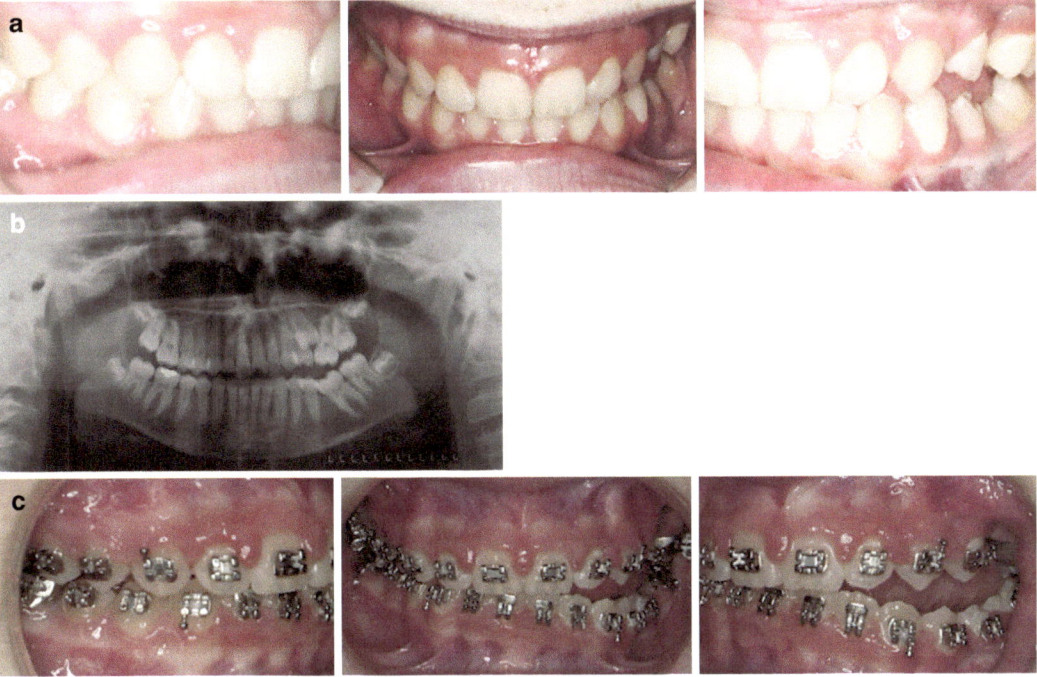

Fig. 2.4 (**a**) Clinical photographs of an 11-year 5-month-old patient who presented for orthodontic treatment and was subsequently diagnosed with ankylosis in the lower left posterior quadrant. (**b**) Pretreatment panoramic radiograph also reveals a blocked-out maxillary left second premolar due to the mesial tipping of the first molar – this was most likely due to the early exfoliation of the second primary molar. This patient did not have history of prior trauma, nor remarkable health history. (**c**) Subsequent treatment with a continuous archwire resulted in worsening of the lateral posterior open bite exemplifying the inability of teeth affected with PFE to respond to orthodontic forces. Several years following treatment, it was determined that the patient harbored a mutation in the *PTH1R* gene similar to her mother and two siblings

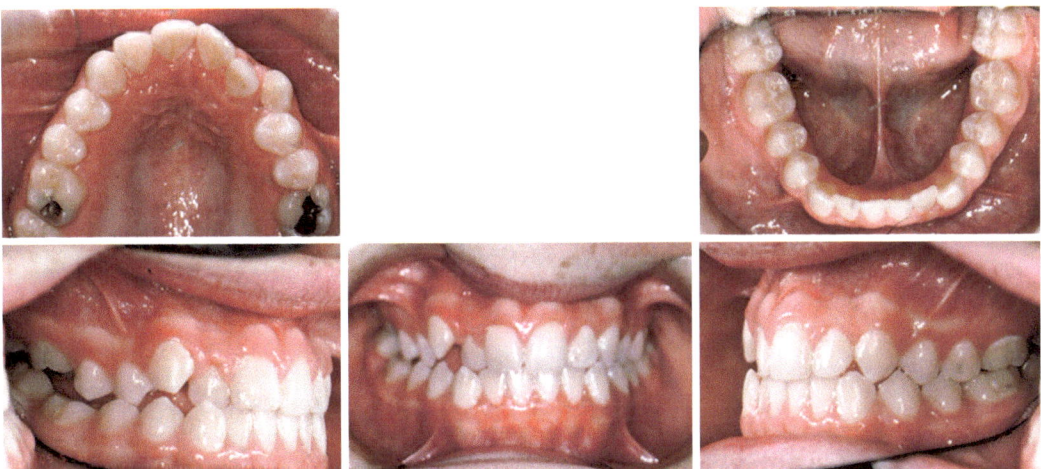

Fig. 2.5 Clinical photographs of a 16-year 5-month-old patient diagnosed with ankylosis of the lower right first molar using "bone sounding methods." This patient did not have history of prior trauma nor remarkable health history. Similar to his siblings, he was later diagnosed with PFE based on the presence of a mutation in the *PTH1R* gene

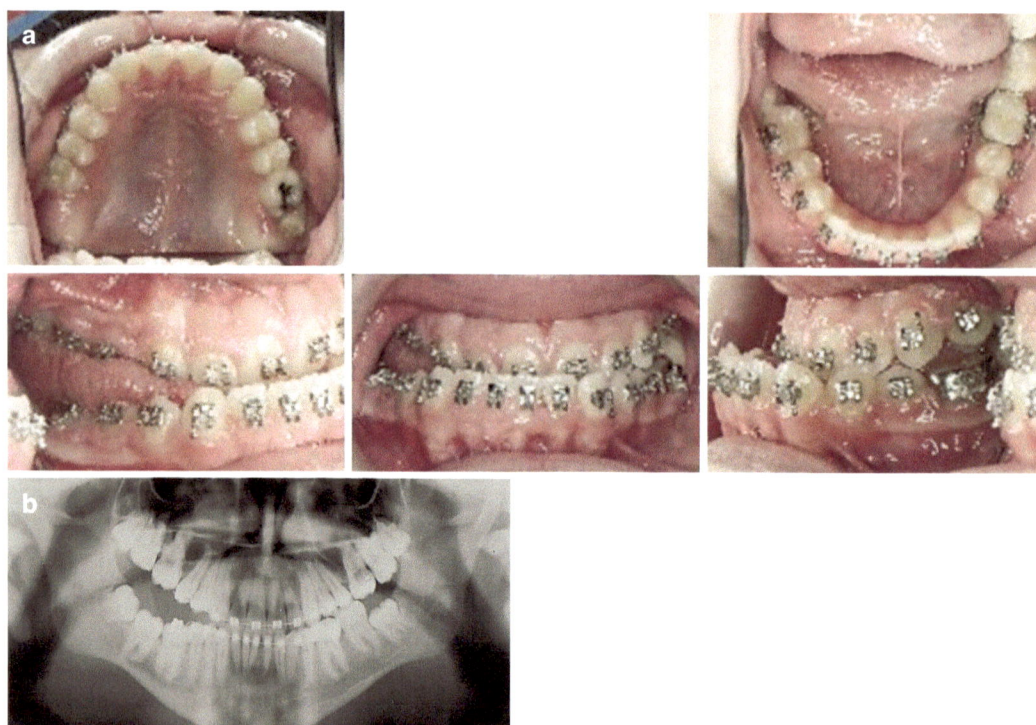

Fig. 2.6 (**a**) Clinical photographs of a 17-year 4-month-old patient undergoing orthodontic treatment primarily for his "underbite." This patient presented with a skeletal Class III malocclusion, severe anterior crossbite, and unilateral posterior crossbite on the right. Treatment with a continuous archwire did not correct the vertical posterior open bite (PFE). (**b**) Panoramic film illustrating eruption failure with a progressive worsening from anterior to posterior. Orthognathic surgical treatment (maxillary advancement) corrected his Class III malocclusion but not his posterior open bite due to PFE. This patient is the sibling of the patient in Figs. 2.4 and 2.5 also harboring a mutation in the *PTH1R* gene

tion of the primary roots may not occur or may be significantly delayed due to the absence of its permanent successor (Fig. 2.7a–c). If the primary tooth ankyloses in a young child [37], it may be overgrown by the surrounding dentition that continues to erupt and the area has further alveolar growth. Teeth that ankylose at a very young age can be completely overgrown by the surrounding dentition and bone creating a complicated surgical problem. If the second primary molar becomes ankylosed, the first permanent molar can tip over the primary molar's occlusal surface causing tipping and space loss. In this instance the primary molar can be built up with a stainless steel crown or by bonding resin to the primary molar occlusal surface to maintain an appropriate contact height with the first permanent molar. In many instances the primary molar that has a permanent successor will undergo normal root resorption and exfoliation requiring no special treatment.

Orthodontic and Surgical Tooth Eruption Therapy

The location of an impacted canine is closely related to the etiology. For instance, a buccally impacted canine is most often a result of crowded dental arches while a palatally impacted canine is often more closely related to a defect in the primary eruption mechanism [36]. Therefore, an approach to manage canines that are buccally impacted may often include extraction of the adjacent first premolars to create space and allow them to erupt into the arch unimpeded. In complete contrast to the blocked-out buccal canine, the palatally impacted canine is more likely to occur with certain features including congenitally absent first premolars, small lateral incisors, enamel hypoplasia, and hypodivergent facial profile [29, 36]. It is essentially always necessary to surgically expose palatally impacted canine teeth and ligate with a bonded pad and chain using orthodontic traction (see Fig. 2.8a–c).

Cleidocranial dysplasia (OMIM #119600) is inherited as an autosomal dominate trait and is caused by mutations in the *RUNX2* gene that is an important signaling protein for normal bone for-

mation and tooth eruption. Affected individuals have short stature, delayed closure of the cranial fontanelles, frontal bossing, supernumerary teeth, and abnormal eruption of the permanent dentition. The phenotype and severity are variable, and in cases of new mutations where there is no family history, it can be difficult to diagnose in children. Treatment will frequently require a team approach involving oral surgery to manage supernumerary teeth and help expose unerupted permanent teeth so they can be orthodontically brought into occlusion (Fig. 2.9a–h). The orthodontist and surgeon should evaluate the affected

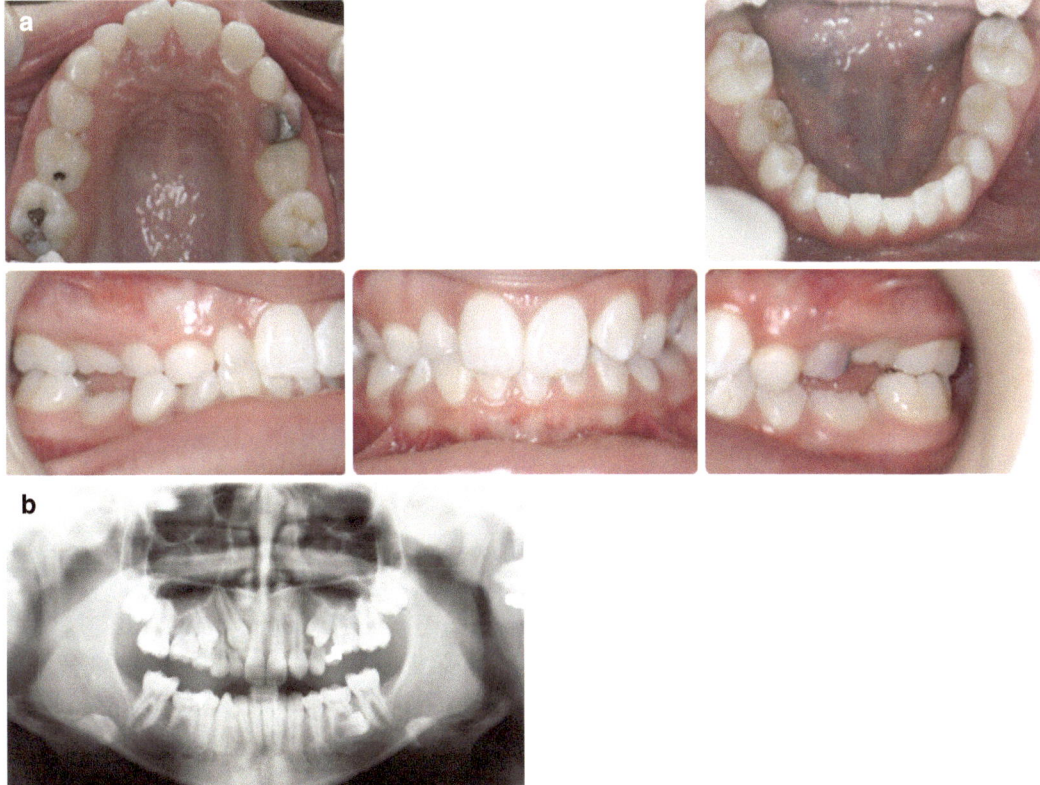

Fig. 2.7 (**a**) Example of ankylosis due to congenitally missing teeth (hypodontia). Initial clinical photographs of a 12-year 6-month-old patient with no history of prior trauma or a familial history of eruption disorders. (**b**) Panoramic radiograph illustrates the ankylosis of primary second molars and maxillary canines associated with congenitally missing maxillary second premolars and laterals as well as an ectopic LL5. The ankylosis is radiographically confirmed due to the infraocclusion of the select teeth, while the adjacent teeth display normal eruption.

(**c**, **d**) Posttreatment clinical records including photographs and panoramic radiograph of the same patient after the extraction of primary canines, primary second molars, and ectopic mandibular left second premolar. The treatment plan included canine substitution to replace maxillary laterals and maintaining spaces for future implants or other prosthetics. After growth is completed, the patient will have the option of either implant/crowns, fixed bridges, or removable partial dentures

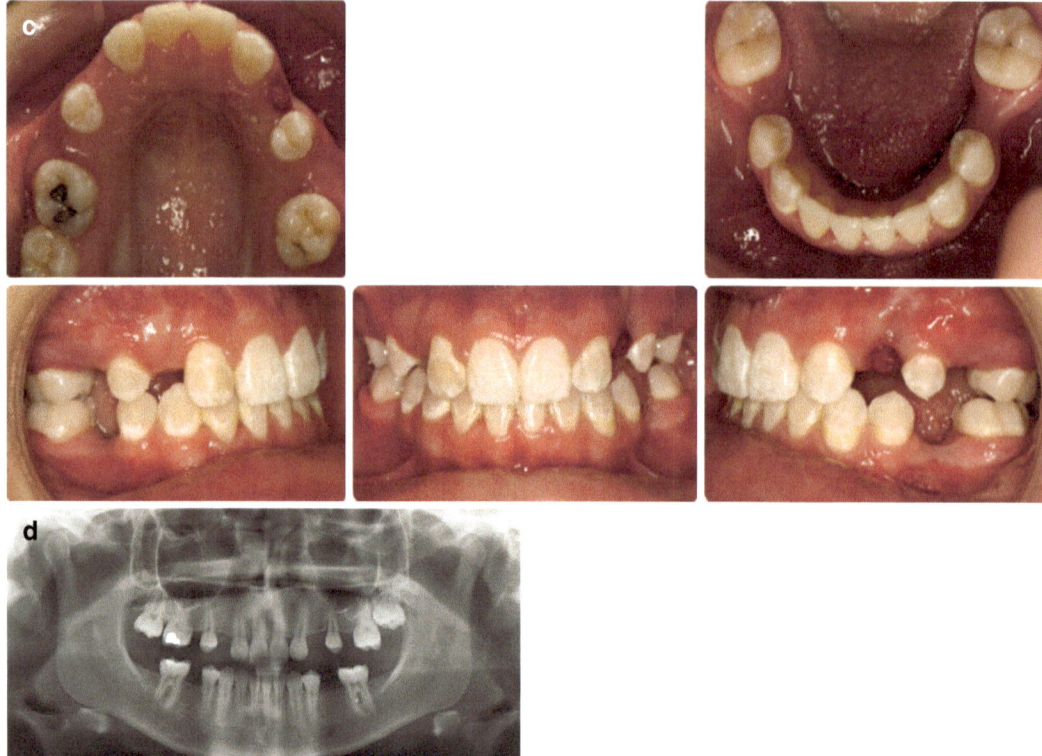

Fig. 2.7 (continued)

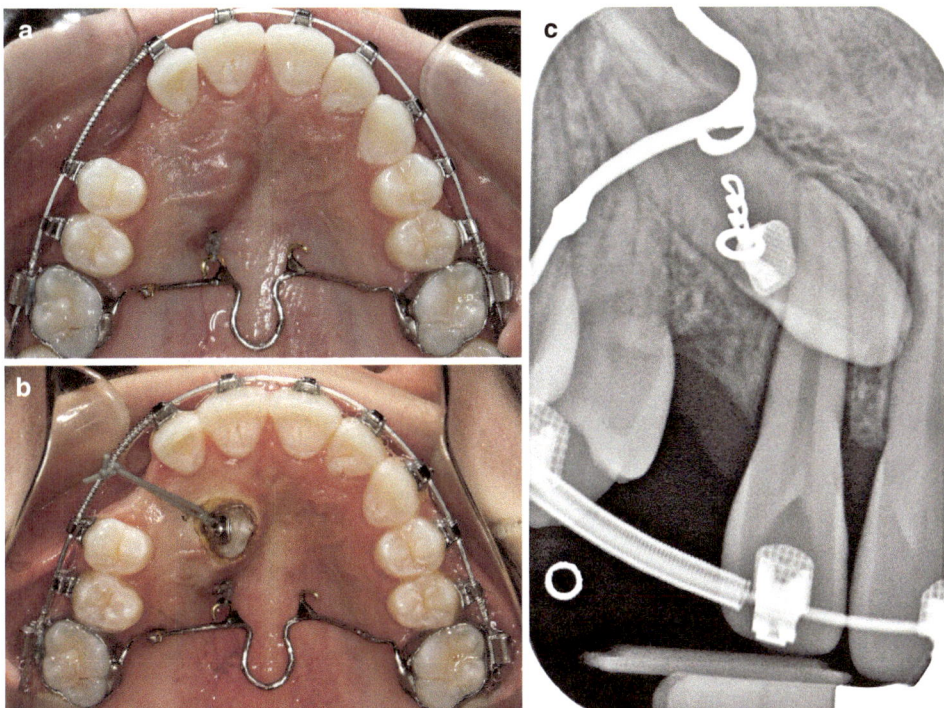

Fig. 2.8 (**a**) Occlusal photograph of an edentulous area where a palatally impacted canine failed to erupt. The patient has the contralateral canine that has erupted into the arch normally. (**b**) The canine was surgically exposed and bonded during the exposure surgery with a linked chain. Subsequent recovering of canine with soft tissue flap resulted in the need to perform soft tissue laser surgery to re-expose the canine. (**c**) A periapical radiograph reveals the canine that is still impacted but ligated to the bonded pad and chain. This clinical scenario will result in a successful result of the canine into the arch

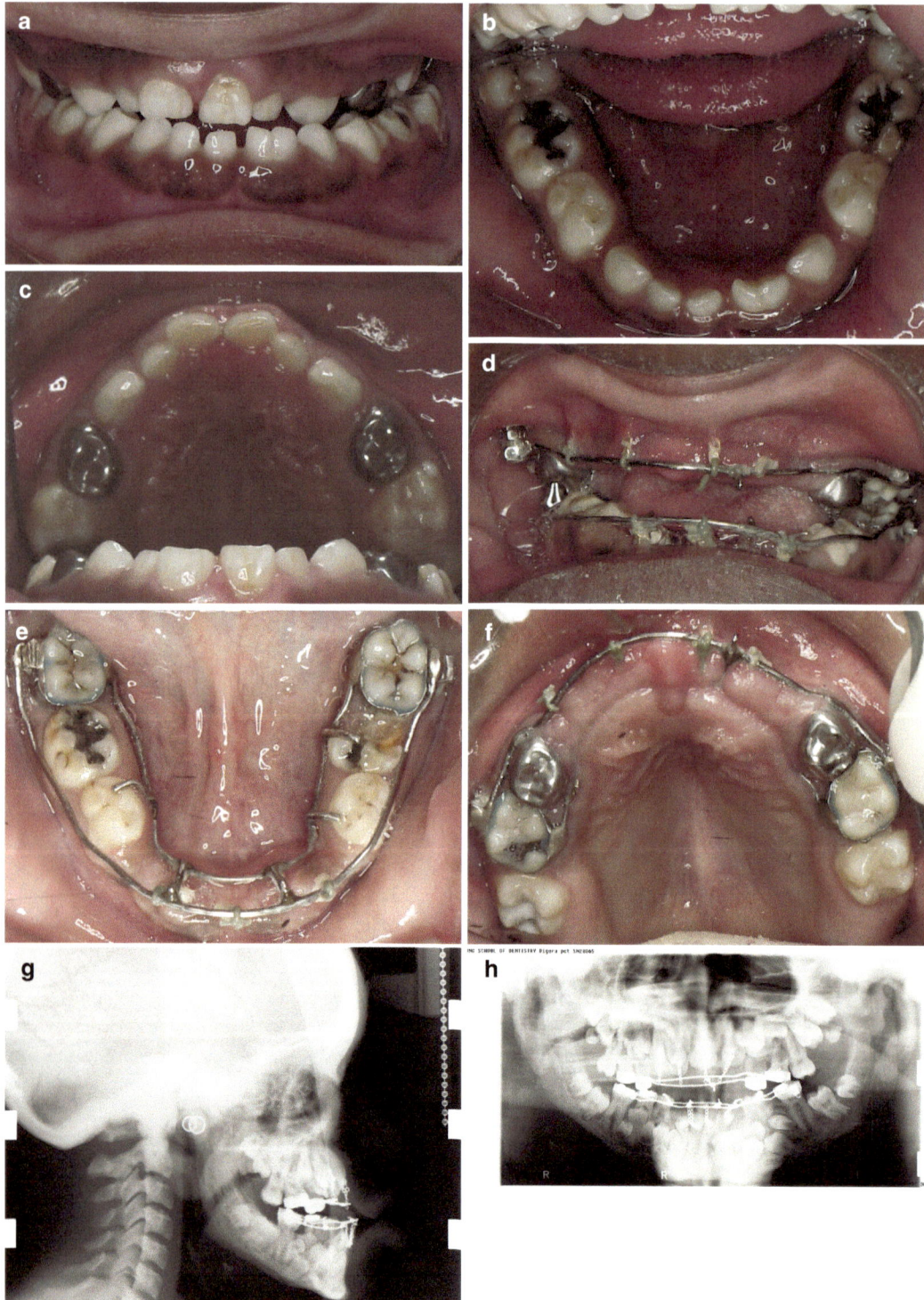

Fig. 2.9 Preoperative photos of a patient with CCD in retained primary dentition before (**a–c**) and after surgical exposures and ligation to a heavy mil arch bar to place traction on the teeth and bring them into occlusion (**d–f**). Radiographic evaluation of the same patient with cephalometric and panoramic films reveals the extent of the unerupted permanent teeth and impaction (**g–h**)

individual to determine what supernumerary teeth are best extracted and when is the optimal time to begin treatment. Some patients will benefit from craniofacial surgery to address the frontal bossing and craniofacial anomalies.

Conclusion

Whether the propulsive force of eruption is created by the bone "pushing" the tooth, or the tooth "pulling" the bone with it, the role of genes critical to the bone remodeling process is evident. Nonetheless, several gaps remain in our understanding of tooth eruption process. Future studies to evaluate additional candidate genes and investigate the role of environmental factors, such as trauma or orthodontic forces, will be essential to completely understand the normal eruption process. Indeed, as suggested by Berkovitz [10], a multifactorial theory (i.e., a combination of environmental factors and the canonical eruption theories) may largely explain the normal process of eruption, but the complex interplay of regulatory factors and environmental cues that contribute to this mechanism is still poorly understood. It is possible that each of the eruption theories above contributes to some portion of the whole process of tooth eruption. For instance, as the Hertwig epithelial root sheath (HERS) moves apically followed by its eventual disintegration and the formation of cementum during root formation (i.e., root elongation theory), it may signal the dental follicle and stellate reticulum cells to secrete mediators of bone remodeling (i.e., dental follicle theory). Mediators secreted from the dental follicle, such as VEGF, also cause angiogenesis and a concomitant increase in the apical tissue pressure propelling the tooth occlusally through the bone (i.e., hydrostatic pressure theory). It is likely that the biological mechanisms above represent portions of the cascade of events that facilitate normal eruption. An alteration of any part of these coordinated signaling events will lead to eruption failure.

From a clinical perspective, the ultimate goal is to understand the normal process of eruption in order to manage those cases of pri-mary and permanent tooth eruption disorders. Primary teeth that fail to erupt fully or that have erupted but are secondarily submerged as the surrounding alveolar bone continues to develop around it are more likely to be ankylosed than permanent teeth with the same fate. However, isolated ankylosis of permanent first molars can be managed by extraction of the offending ankylosed tooth allowing for normal eruption of the second and third molars. A failure of the second and third molars to erupt fully would be pathognomonic for PFE. A hallmark of PFE is the response of affected teeth to orthodontic force; orthodontic force *will not* result in eruption of the affected tooth but will in fact lead to ankylosis of the affected teeth or intrusion of the adjacent teeth. Finally, another critical clue to diagnosing and managing cases of eruption failure is that the genetic association with *PTH1R* confirms the importance of determining a good family history. The American Society of Human Genetics suggested that taking a family history represents the gold standard in the diagnosis of and management of medical (and by extension, dental) disorders [35]. This judicious combination of clinical, biological, and genetic factors will change the way we have practiced in the past but will lead to the successful diagnosis and treatment of nearly all clinical disorders in the not so distant future.

References

1. Proffit WR. Contemporary Orthodontics. 5th ed. Elsevier 2013. St Louis, Missouri.
2. Helfrich MH. Osteoclast diseases and dental abnormalities. Arch Oral Biol. 2005;50(2):115–22. Eighth international conference on Tooth Morphogenesis and Differentiation.
3. Proffit WR, Vig KW. Primary failure of eruption: a possible cause of posterior open-bite. Am J Orthod. 1981;80(2):173–90.
4. Frazier-Bowers SA, Simmons D, Wright JT, et al. Primary eruption failure and *PTH1R*: the importance of a genetic diagnosis for orthodontic treatment planning. Am J Orthod Dentofac Orthop. 2010;137(160).1–7.
5. Wise GE, King GJ. Mechanisms of tooth eruption and orthodontic tooth movement. J Dent Res. 2008;87:414–34.

6. Suri L, Gagari E, Vastardis H. Delayed tooth eruption: pathogenesis, diagnosis, and treatment. A literature review. Am J Orthod Dentofac Orthop. 2004;126: 432–45.
7. Frazier-Bowers SA, Koehler KE, Ackerman JL, et al. Primary failure of eruption: further characterization of a rare eruption disorder. Am J Orthod Dentofac Orthop. 2007;131(5):578.e1–11.
8. Decker E, Stellzig-Eisenhauer A, Fiebig βS, et al. PTHR1 loss-of-function mutations in familial, non-syndromic primary failure of tooth eruption. Am J Hum Genet. 2008;83(6):781–6.
9. Bjork A. The use of metallic implants in the study of facial growth in children: method and application. Am J Phys Anthropol. 1968;29(2):243–54.
10. Berkovitz BK. How teeth erupt. Dent Update. 1990; 17(5):206–10.
11. Ten Cate AR, Nanci A. Physiologic tooth movement: eruption and shedding. In: Nanci A, editor. Oral histology: development, structure and function. 7th ed. Toronto: Mosby; 2008. p. 268–88.
12. Cahill DR, Marks Jr SC. Tooth eruption: evidence for the central role of the dental follicle. J Oral Pathol. 1980;9(4):189–200.
13. Marks Jr SC, Cahill DR. Regional control by the dental follicle of alterations in alveolar bone metabolism during tooth eruption. J Oral Pathol. 1987;16(4):164–9.
14. Wise GE, Frazier-Bowers S, D'Souza RN. Cellular, molecular, and genetic determinants of tooth eruption. Crit Rev Oral Biol Med. 2002;13(4):323–34. Review.
15. Beertsen W, Hoeben KA. Movement of fibroblasts in the periodontal ligament of the mouse incisor is related to eruption. J Dent Res. 1987;66:1006–10.
16. Kasugai S, Suzuki S, Shibata S, Yasui S, Amano H, Ogura H. Measurements of the isometric contractile forces generated by dog periodontal ligament fibroblasts in vitro. Arch Oral Biol. 1990;35:597–601.
17. Berkovitz BK, Migdalski A, Solomon M. The effect of the lathyritic agent aminoacetonitrile on the unimpeded eruption rate in normal and root-resected rat lower incisors. Arch Oral Biol. 1972;17(12):1755–63.
18. Gron AM. Prediction of tooth emergence. J Dent Res. 1962;41:573–85.
19. Moorrees CFA, Fanning EA, Hunt EEJ. Age variation of formation stages for ten permanent teeth. J Dent Res. 1963;42:1490–502.
20. Berkovitz BK. The effect of root transection and partial root resection on the unimpeded eruption rate of the rat incisor. Arch Oral Biol. 1971;16(9):1033–42.
21. Wise GE. Cellular and molecular basis of tooth eruption. Orthod Craniofacial Res. 2009;12(2):67–73.
22. Van Hassel HJ, McMinn RG. Pressure differential favouring tooth eruption in the dog. Arch Oral Biol. 1972;17(1):183–90.
23. Cheek CC, Paterson RL, Proffit WR. Response of erupting human second premolars to blood flow changes. Arch Oral Biol. 2002;47:851–8.
24. Yao S, Pan F, Wise GE. Chronological gene expression of parathyroid hormone-related protein (PTHrP) in the stellate reticulum of the rat: implications for tooth eruption. Arch Oral Biol. 2007;52(3):228–32.
25. Castaneda B, Simon Y, Jacques J, Hess E, Choi Y-W, Blin-Wakkach C, Mueller C, Berdal A, Lézot F. Bone resorption control of tooth eruption and root morphogenesis: involvement of the receptor activator of NF-κB (RANK). J Cell Physiol. 2011;226: 74–85.
26. Frazier-Bowers SA, Puranik CP, Mahaney MC. The etiology of eruption disorders – further evidence of a 'genetic paradigm.'. Semin Orthod. 2010;16(3):180–5.
27. Baccetti T. A controlled study of associated dental anomalies. Angle Orthod. 1998;68(3):267–74.
28. Pirinen S, Arte S, Apajalahti S. Palatal displacement of canine is genetic and related to congenital absence of teeth. J Dent Res. 1996;75(10):1742–6.
29. Peck S, Peck L, Kataja M. The palatally displaced canine as a dental anomaly of genetic origin. Angle Orthod. 1994;64(4):249–56.
30. Rhoads SG, Hendricks HM, Frazier-Bowers SA. Establishing the diagnostic criteria for eruption disorders based on genetic and clinical data. Am J Orthod Dentofac Orthop. 2013;144(2):194–202.
31. Biederman W. Etiology and treatment of and treatment of tooth ankylosis. Am J Orthod. 1962;48:670–84.
32. Raghoebar GM, Boering G, Vissink A. Clinical, radiographic and histological characteristics of secondary retention of permanent molars. J Dent. 1991; 19(3):164–70.
33. Thilander B, Myrberg N. The prevalence of malocclusion in Swedish schoolchildren. Scand J Dent Res. 1973;81(1):12–21.
34. Magnusson TE. Prevalence of hypodontia and malformations of permanent teeth in Iceland. Community Dent Oral Epidemiol. 1977;5(4):173–8.
35. American Society of Human Genetics. New research validates clinical use of family health history as the 'gold standard' for assessing personal disease risk [Press release]. 2010. Retrieved from http://www. ashg.org/pdf/PR_FamilyHealthHistory_110510.pdf
36. Baccetti T, Leonard M, Guintini V. Distally displaced premolars: a dental anomaly associated with palatally displaced canines. Am J Orthod Dentofacial Orthop. 2010;138:318–22.
37. Tieu LD, Walker SL, Major MP, Flores-Mir C. Management of ankylosed primary molars with premolar successors: a systematic review. J Am Dent Assoc. 2013;144(6):602–11.
38. Silvestrini Biavati A, Signori A, Castaldo A, Matarese G, Migliorati M. Incidence and distribution of deciduous molar ankylosis, a longitudinal study. Eur J Paediatr Dent. 2011;12(3):175–8.
39. Kurol J. Infraocclusion of primary molars: an epidemiologic and familial study. Community Dent Oral Epidemiol. 1981;9(2):94–102.
40. Shalish M, Peck S, Wasserstein A, Peck L. Increased occurrence of dental anomalies associated with infraocclusion of deciduous molars. Angle Orthod. 2010;80(3):440–5. doi:10.2319/062609-358.1.

Conditions Associated with Premature Exfoliation of Primary Teeth or Delayed Eruption of Permanent Teeth

3

Michael Milano

Abstract

Although exfoliation of primary teeth and the subsequent eruption of the permanent successors usually occur in a systematic fashion, there are numerous conditions that can impact this developmental process. These conditions can be broadly grouped into the following categories:

1. Environmental factors
2. Genetic conditions
3. Endocrine conditions
4. Immunological conditions
5. Gestational factors

The mechanisms through which these conditions affect tooth eruption are diverse, and the diagnosis and management can be quite challenging for the oral health-care provider. These factors and conditions will be examined and material provided on clinical presentation and treatment options. Finally, where possible, each hereditary condition is identified by its OMIM number so that the reader can easily obtain additional information.

Introduction

During development of the human dentition, the 20 primary teeth emerge providing the infant and child with a masticatory apparatus and serving as a template that helps guide in the permanent dentition. Thus exfoliation of primary teeth is an expected and normally a fairly predictable process. Although the order of exfoliation commonly follows a set pattern, there can be variation in the timing of exfoliation of a year or more. This variation is usually not considered abnormal as long as it reflects the individual child's dental development. In general, mandibular teeth exfoliate prior to maxillary teeth, usually from the anterior to posterior regions, the exception being the maxillary canines. This process occurs earlier in girls than boys [1]. However, primary teeth that exfoliate early, outside of the child's pattern of dental development, can be a concern as this could reflect an underlying local or systemic pathology.

M. Milano
Department of Pediatric Dentistry,
School of Dentistry, University of North Carolina,
Chapel Hill, NC, USA
e-mail: Michael_Milano@unc.edu.

J.T. Wright (ed.), *Craniofacial and Dental Developmental Defects: Diagnosis and Management*,
DOI 10.1007/978-3-319-13057-6_3, © Springer International Publishing Switzerland 2015

This chapter will examine some of these underlying conditions in a format that is meant to provide the practitioner with a straightforward approach to diagnosis and management. It is important to note that many of the conditions discussed in this chapter occur with an underlying medical condition. This necessitates that diagnosis, and often treatment, will include both medical and dental professionals [2].

The format of this chapter has been chosen so as to provide the reader with a logical approach to information gathering and diagnosis, the critical first step in appropriate management. The conditions in this chapter are presented in three formats. Each condition is described in a traditional text format. In addition, each is also listed in a table format allowing the reader to reach a tentative diagnosis by starting with a clinical presentation. Finally clinical photos are included as an additional method of identifying the diagnostic challenge facing the practitioner.

Premature Exfoliation of Primary Teeth

Environmental Factors

There are many environmental factors that affect tooth development as discussed in the chapters covering the topics of hypodontia and enamel and dentin anomalies. Similarly, there are different environmental factors that can influence the process of tooth exfoliation. Premature exfoliation of primary teeth can challenge the clinician to determine whether the etiology is the result of environmental, systemic illness, or hereditary factors.

Acrodynia
Acrodynia, also known as "pink disease," is a rare condition that is seen with hypersensitive children when using medications or creams with a mercury base [3, 4]. Clinical features include fever, severe sweating, anorexia, listlessness, irritability, tachycardia, hypertension, photophobia, and a desquamation of the palms of the hands and the soles of the feet resulting in the "pink skin" [1, 3].

Oral findings include inflammation and ulceration of the mucous membranes. In addition, hypersalivation has also been reported. Premature exfoliation of primary teeth can occur secondary to a loss of alveolar bone [3].

Given the extensive physical signs and symptoms of this condition, diagnosis is likely to occur prior to presentation to the dentist with treatment being palliative in nature.

Autoextraction
Although autoextraction is not a common occurrence, it can be seen associated with certain conditions in which individuals demonstrate self-injurious behaviors. These conditions include congenital indifference to pain syndrome and Lesch-Nyhan syndrome, among others [5]. This self-injurious behavior can manifest itself intraorally as soft tissue lacerations, ulcers, and premature tooth loss via autoextraction [5]. Armstrong and Matt (1999) reported a case of autoextraction in an autistic patient who can have hyposensitivity to pain and in one case report the person with autism removed seven permanent teeth over the course of several months [5]. Unfortunately treatment options are extremely limited in most instances.

Genetic Conditions

Chediak-Higashi Syndrome
Chediak-Higashi syndrome (OMIM #214500) is an autosomal recessive trait, with a variable age of onset, caused by mutations in the lysosomal trafficking regulator gene that results in neutropenia and abnormal susceptibility to infection [1]. Clinical features include respiratory and skin infections. In addition, ocular features are also commonly seen, including both strabismus and nystagmus [1]. Dental findings include an early onset and severe destruction of the periodontium which results in significant mobility of the teeth. This periodontal destruction is very commonly associated with severe gingivitis [1].

Diagnosis of Chediak-Higashi syndrome is likely to have been made prior to the patient presenting for a dental evaluation. Dental treatment would be palliative, addressing the patient's symptoms. Bailleul-Forestier et al. [6] reported a case of a 12-year-old female with Chediak-Higashi syndrome who presented with significant periodontal involvement. The authors reported that following appropriate treatment intervention, which included initial periodontal therapy, frequent recalls, patient compliance, and continuous long-term antibiotic therapy, the patient was able to maintain periodontal health over a 9-year follow-up period [6]. A medical referral should be made if necessary as these individuals are susceptible to recurrent infections and prolonged bleeding time [6].

Singleton-Merten Syndrome

Singleton-Merten syndrome (OMIM #182250) is a multiple system disorder that is inherited as an autosomal dominant trait [1]. Because of this multisystem involvement and with death occurring between 4 and 18 years of age, it would likely be diagnosed based on clinical features rather than dental features.

Clinical features of Singleton-Merten include skeletal deformities of the hands and feet along with subluxation of joints, ruptured ligaments, muscle weakness, short stature, and osteoporosis. Idiopathic calcification of the aortic arch and valve is a commonly seen cardiac feature. Glaucoma and infertility have also been reported [1, 7].

Dental abnormalities affect both the primary and permanent dentitions with early loss of both dentitions [1, 7]. The primary dentition may also demonstrate delayed eruption and immature root formation. This, along with acute root resorption and alveolar bone loss, results in the mobility and early loss of the primary dentition [1, 7]. Management of the dentition is palliative.

Coffin-Lowry Syndrome

Children with Coffin-Lowry syndrome (OMIM #303600), an X-linked inherited condition caused by mutations in a growth factor-related gene [1, 8], present with intellectual disabilities and skeletal anomalies [1, 8–10]. These children present with classic facial features related to the persistent anterior fontanel (Fig. 3.1). Thick hands, extensible joints, and hypotonia along

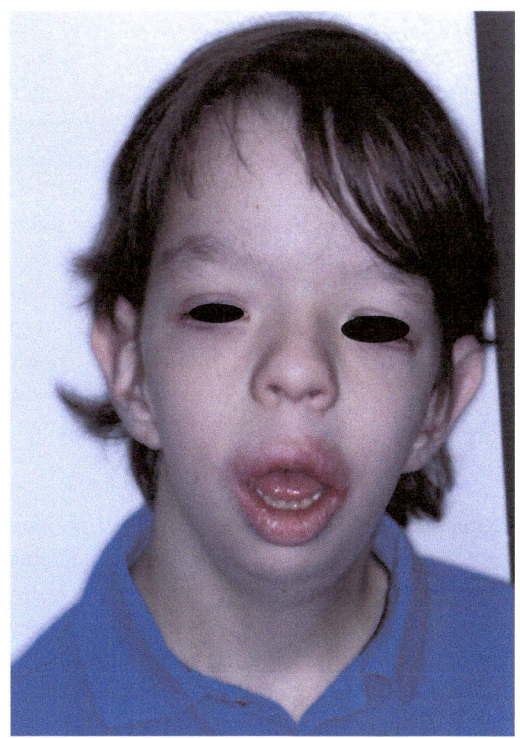

Fig. 3.1 Typical facial appearance of Coffin-Lowry syndrome

with sensorineural hearing loss are all common features [1, 8–10].

Oral features associated with Coffin-Lowry syndrome include both soft and hard tissues. Soft tissue features include a furrowed tongue and thick lips [8]. Also noteworthy are mandibular prognathism, high vaulted palate, microdontia, and premature exfoliation of primary teeth [1, 8–10]. These primary teeth exfoliate without root resorption since the pathological mechanism appears to be hypoplastic cementum [10].

The presentation of dental findings may aid in the diagnosis but the spectrum of clinical features make it likely the diagnosis would be made prior to the presentation to the dental professional. Treatment includes palliative care with extraction of mobile symptomatic teeth along with aggressive oral hygiene practices [8].

Hajdu-Cheney Syndrome

Hajdu-Cheney syndrome (OMIM #102500) is a rare progressive disorder of bone metabolism which results in a dissolution of the hand's and feet's terminal phalanges [11, 12]. It demonstrates an autosomal dominant pattern of inheritance due to mutations in the NOTCH2 gene that is an important regulator of gene expression. Hajdu-Cheney syndrome is characterized by a variable cluster of clinical manifestations affecting skeletal and other tissues [1, 11, 12].

The clinical features of this syndrome are quite obvious. In addition to the bony dissolution in the hands and feet, patients with Hajdu-Cheney also demonstrate joint laxity, short stature, scoliosis, kyphosis, and multiple osteolytic lesions [1, 11, 12].

These children also present with characteristic facial features. The craniofacial features, although not pathognomonic, are relatively distinctive. These features include an elongated skull with a widened sella turcica, absence of a frontal sinus, small chin, and a dolichocephalic appearance [11, 12]. Coarse hair, thick eyebrows, and clubbing of the fingers are also seen [11].

Oral features in Hajdu-Cheney include both hard and soft tissue pathology. Inflammation of the gingiva with bleeding on probing is present. An underlying periodontitis with atrophy of the alveolar bone also occurs [11]. The hard tissue changes that have been reported include hypoplastic roots along with structural changes in the cementum and dentin which results in premature tooth loss [11, 12].

Ehlers-Danlos Syndrome

Ehlers-Danlos (OMIM #130090) represents a group of inherited disorders that are caused by mutations in the genes that code for different collagens and a variety of other proteins. Patients with Ehlers-Danlos demonstrate hyperextensible skin along with hypermobility of the joints of their digits [1, 13, 14]. The underlying pathological mechanism of this condition is related to a disordered collagen metabolism. Multiple subtypes have been recognized resulting in a prevalence of 1 in 5,000 live births for this autosomal dominant condition [1, 13, 14].

The reported dental changes are also related to the abnormal collagen metabolism and vary between the different subtypes. This disordered metabolism is thought to result in enhanced resorption of the crest of the alveolar bone and apices of the roots [13]. In addition, fragility of the oral mucosa and blood vessels, along with the concomitant aggressive periodontitis, results in severe alveolar bone loss with related tooth loss. Inflamed gingiva is also readily seen [13].

The primary goal of the indicated dental treatment is to control the disease and subsequent tooth loss. Unfortunately targeting oral hygiene alone does not produce enough of an impact to control the loss of clinical attachment which leads to the premature exfoliation of the teeth. It has also been reported that orthodontic treatment can exacerbate this bone loss [13, 14].

Papillon-Lefevre Syndrome

Papillon-Lefevre syndrome (OMIM #245000) is caused by mutations in the cathepsin C gene that codes for a protein with important function in immune cells. Perhaps the most striking clinical feature of this syndrome, and something that is diagnostic for this condition, is the hyperkeratosis of the palms of the hands and the soles of the feet (Fig. 3.2a, b) [1, 3, 15–18]. This rare genetic disorder follows an autosomal recessive pattern of inheritance and is seen equally in males and females with an incidence of one to four per million live births having been reported [1, 15–18].

The onset of the associated dental changes coincides with the eruption of the primary teeth and with the start of the hyperkeratosis [17]. The premature loss of teeth, which can affect both dentitions, is related to the severe periodontitis and bone loss. The gingiva is hyperemic and edematous with deep periodontal pocketing [15, 18]. The teeth become progressively more mobile resulting in discomfort with eating [16]. Dental radiographs taken on these patients demonstrate generalized alveolar bone destruction associated with the primary dentition [16].

Although a diagnosis of Papillon-Lefevre syndrome can be made histologically from biopsies from the skin of the hands and feet, it is usually made based on the clinical presentation and

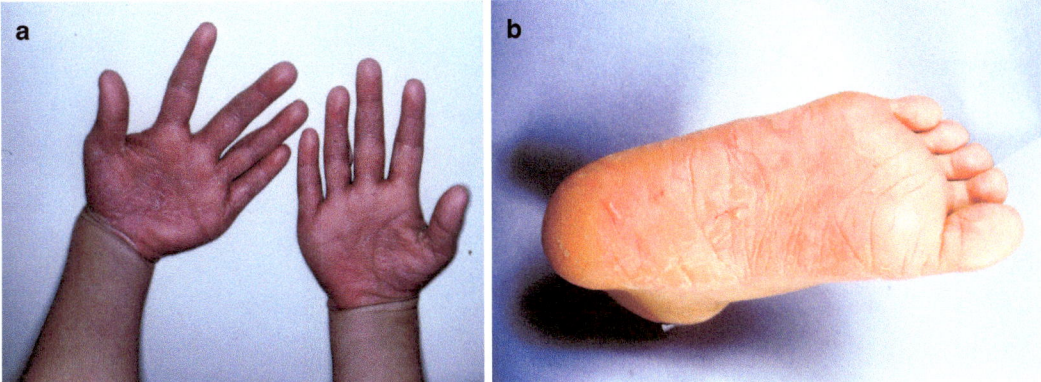

Fig. 3.2 (**a**) and (**b**) Palmoplantar hyperkeratosis as seen in Papillon-Lefevre syndrome

genetic testing [18]. Clinically, the three features required for a diagnosis are [18]:

1. Autosomal recessive inheritance
2. Palmoplantar hyperkeratosis
3. Loss of the primary and permanent dentitions

A multifaceted treatment approach is required for Papillon-Lefevre syndrome. Treatment usually consists of four components: (1) aggressive professional in-office care (2), treatment of involved symptomatic teeth (3), excellent home care and oral hygiene, and (4) antibiotics. In-office care includes periodontal debridement along with scaling and root planing. Extraction of hopeless teeth should also be performed. In some cases early full-mouth extraction of the primary teeth is recommended so that the permanent teeth can erupt into a healthier environment [3, 17].

Outside of the dental office, treatment includes methods for aggressive local plaque control [15]. In addition antibiotics are sometimes used. The use of both broad-spectrum antibiotics and those aimed at specific identified organisms has been reported in the literature [3, 15, 17, 18]. Early treatment is important since it may aid in the retention of the permanent dentition [1].

Cherubism

Cherubism (OMIM #118400) is a rare condition that has an onset of between 2 and 4 years of age [1]. It is inherited as an autosomal dominant trait and it is known to have a highly variable expressivity [1, 3]. This is a fibroosseous condition characterized by osteoclastic degeneration of the upper and lower jaws followed by development of fibrous masses.

The two most common clinical features give rise to the typical facial appearance seen with cherubism. Involvement of the maxilla with displacement of the globes along with the bilateral mandibular swelling yields the characteristic facial appearance of these children [3]. These symmetrical mandibular swellings usually increase in size until puberty and stabilize and often regress after that [1, 18].

Radiographically these mandibular swellings present as multilocular radiolucent cystic lesions which can also be seen in the ribs [1, 3, 19]. These multilocular cysts can impact the overlying dentition (Fig. 3.3). They can cause displacement of the primary and permanent dentition. As these teeth become more mobile, there is resultant pain with the teeth eventually exfoliating. In some cases exfoliation of the primary dentition can occur as early as 22 months [1, 3, 19].

A diagnosis of cherubism is based on a combination of all findings including clinical, radiographic, and histological. A family history can also help with the diagnosis [19]. Treatment will vary depending on the needs of the affected individual. Surgical reduction of the bony lesions can be accomplished if the child is having psychosocial issues due to their appearance. While the lesions tend to regress after puberty, lesion regression may not occur until much later in life. Surgical treatment coupled with autoge-

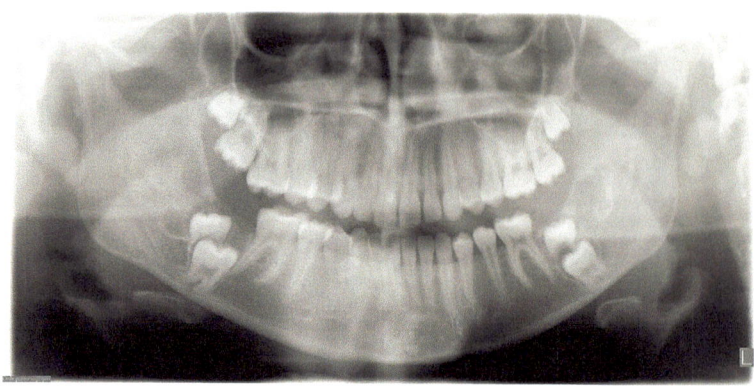

Fig. 3.3 Panoramic radiograph of a patient with cherubism. Multilocular lesions are evident in the mandible bilaterally

nous bone grafting and postoperative treatment to reduce osteoclast activities also have been reported [20].

Dental prostheses can be made to assist with mastication when teeth are lost due to progression of the fibroosseous lesions that can result in tooth displacement and loss.

Endocrine Conditions

Hypophosphatemia

Hypophosphatemia or hypophosphatemic rickets is an abnormality of renal tubular transport of phosphate that can present in various forms. These include X-linked (OMIM #307800), the autosomal dominant vitamin D-resistant forms (OMIM #193100), and the autosomal recessive inherited trait (OMIM #241520) [3, 21]. Clinical features often become evident by the second year of life and include short stature and boxed legs [3, 21].

Dentally these children have thin hypomineralized enamel along with large pulp chambers and high pulp horns which can result in pulp exposures even in the absence of dental caries. These pulp exposures can lead to spontaneous dental abscesses that result in bone loss and the early loss of primary teeth [3, 21].

Diagnosis will often be made by a physician prior to any dental examination. However, dental radiographs will indicate the enamel and pulp chamber changes already mentioned. In addition, changes in the trabeculation of the alveolar bone along with abnormal or absent lamina dura can be observed radiographically [3].

Treatment will depend upon the patient's presentation. Patients will often be given vitamin D analogs and phosphate supplements to improve tooth and bone mineralization. Pulp therapy followed by full-coverage crowns is often indicated along with extraction of abscessed teeth. Despite these different interventions and treatment, dental management in patients with severe dental manifestations is challenging, and outcomes of these therapeutic approaches are not well documented.

Hyperthyroidism

Hyperthyroidism (OMIM #275000) is an autosomal dominant condition that results in an autoimmune reaction. Antibodies to the thyrotropin receptors are generated which results in an overproduction of thyroid hormone via a physiological feedback cycle. In the presence of preexisting periodontal bone loss, an increase in circulating thyroid hormone will result in an increase in the number of bone resorbing cells which in turn results in an increase in bone maturation and turnover. This accounts for the alveolar bone loss, premature exfoliation of the primary dentition, and an associated accelerated eruption of the permanent dentition [1, 22].

This increase in circulating thyroid hormone is also the etiological factor for the clinical features seen in hyperthyroidism. These include hyperactivity and emotional disturbances [1, 22]. Diagnosis would be based on blood work which would show an increased level of circulating thyroid hormone, and dental treatment would be based on the patient's symptoms.

Hypophosphatasia

Hypophosphatasia is characterized by improper mineralization of bone secondary to defective or deficient alkaline phosphatase [1, 3, 15, 23]. This inheritable condition has multiple forms with different modes of inheritance including autosomal recessive and autosomal dominant transmission [1, 3, 24].

Although the three different forms of hypophosphatasia vary in prognosis, in general the earlier the disease manifests itself, the increased severity of the disease [1, 3]. The phenotypes for these forms vary from the mildest with premature loss of deciduous teeth to severe abnormalities of bone with neonatal death [15].

The three forms, which are based on age of onset, are infantile, juvenile or childhood, and adult [3, 25]. These three types of hypophosphatasia have historically been delineated based on the time of diagnosis and level of severity [3]:

1. Infantile: autosomal recessive, usually lethal (OMIM #241500)
2. Juvenile (or childhood): autosomal recessive, milder form (OMIM #241510)
3. Adult: autosomal dominant, mildest (OMIM #146300)

The predominant dental finding in hypophosphatasia is mobility and premature loss of the primary teeth, most often the mandibular anterior [3, 25]. This tooth loss is usually spontaneous with the exfoliation being associated with a loss of alveolar bone along with defective or hypoplastic cementum (Fig. 3.4) [1, 3]. Alkaline phosphatase is critical for normal development of mineralized tissues, and hypophosphatasia results in abnormal cementoblast function and the cell's ability to regulate pyrophosphates critical for normal tissue formation and mineralization during cementogenesis. This defective cementum results in a weakened tooth to alveolar bone attachment which in turn leads to the loss of the primary dentition [15]. This tooth loss is associated with minimal gingival inflammation and minimal plaque buildup (Fig. 3.5) [1, 14].

Since the teeth are usually affected in the order that they are formed, teeth that are formed earlier are the teeth that are usually involved; this includes the mandibular anterior primary teeth

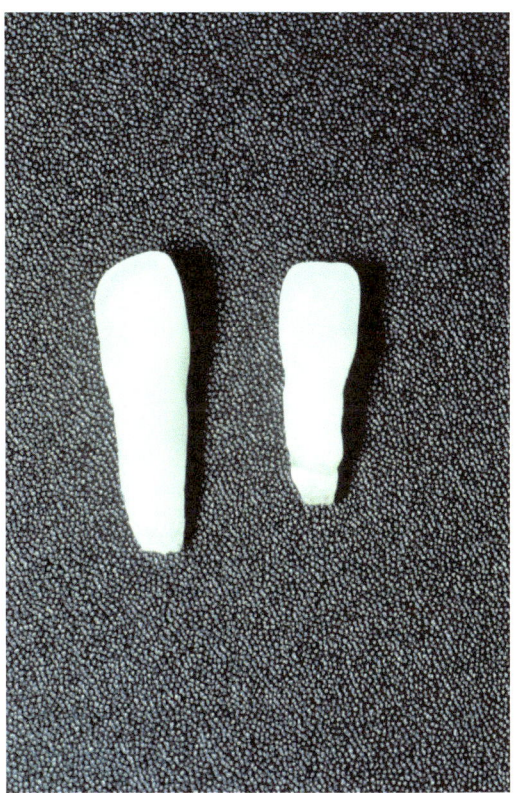

Fig. 3.4 Prematurely exfoliated teeth as seen in hypophosphatasia

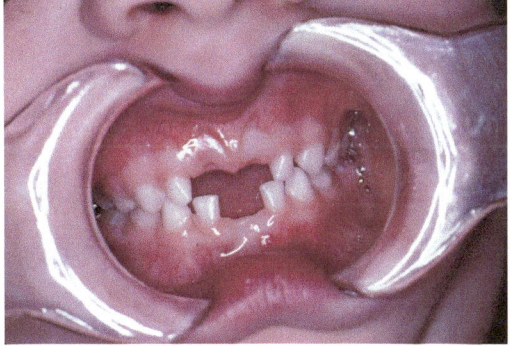

Fig. 3.5 Minimal inflammation seen in the area of prematurely exfoliated teeth in a child with hypophosphatasia

[15]. It should be noted that posterior teeth can also exfoliate prematurely [23]. Additional dental findings that have been reported include enamel hypoplasia, enlarged pulp chambers and root canals, bulbous crowns, and delayed dentin formation [23, 24].

Hypophosphatasia can be diagnosed in two different ways. Laboratory tests can be used to determine the level of serum alkaline phosphatase. In hypophosphatasia a deficient serum and bone alkaline phosphatase activity is found [3, 15, 23]. An additional method of diagnosis involves histological examination of the cementum. Histological samples will indicate hypoplasia of the cementum to the point of a virtual absence of it, resulting in exfoliation of the primary dentition prior to root resorption [1, 23].

Recently, Whyte et al. [26] reported the results of a multinational, open-label study of treatment with ENB0040, a recombinant human tissue nonspecific alkaline phosphatase (TNSALP; 171760) coupled to a deca-aspartate motif for targeting, an enzyme replacement therapy for infantile hypophosphatasia. In this study 11 infants or young children with life-threatening hypophosphatasia were enrolled. Improvement in developmental milestones and pulmonary function along with the healing of bony changes was noted in nine patients after 6 months of therapy [26]. Management of this condition has until now been palliative in nature, aimed at the relief of symptoms often by the use of nonsteroidal anti-inflammatory medications [15, 23]. Dental management emphasizes thorough prevention and oral hygiene regimens [23]. Although the prognosis for the affected primary teeth is poor, it is good for the permanent teeth as these are usually uninvolved [23]. It is not yet clear what the potential benefit of enzyme replacement therapy might be for the dental manifestations and timing of treatment may be problematic unless therapy is initiated during root formation so cementogenesis can progress normally.

Immunological Conditions

Prepubertal Periodontitis

With an onset by 4 years of age, prepubertal periodontitis exists in both localized and generalized forms [1]. The localized form presents with little gingival involvement, demonstrating few signs of inflammation [1]. In the generalized form, severe acute gingival inflammation and recession are noted around all of the primary teeth [1]. The destruction

of alveolar bone in prepubertal periodontitis is more rapid than what is seen with the adult form [1].

The tooth loss exhibited in prepubertal periodontitis can be mistaken for that associated with hypophosphatasia. However in prepubertal periodontitis, which in girls is one of the most common reasons for premature exfoliation of the primary teeth, the children are seropositive for *Actinobacillus actinomycetemcomitans* [1].

Leukocyte Adhesion Deficiency

This rare autosomal recessive disorder (OMIM #612840) is characterized by a defect associated with the white blood cells which results in a defect of their phagocytic function [13, 27–29]. The resultant defective or deficient surface protein causes poor leukocyte migration to the site of infection [15]. This leads to the impaired phagocytic function of the leukocytes and a subsequent increased risk of infection, including periodontitis [15, 22].

The clinical features of leukocyte adhesion deficiency are all related to this impaired leukocytic function. These children present with recurrent fungal and bacterial infections with impaired wound healing. Recurrent infections of the skin and otitis media are commonly seen along with necrotic infections of the gastrointestinal tract and mucous membranes [15, 27–29]. These skin infections are often without the formation of any purulence [29].

The pathologies within the oral cavity are all a function of a severe chronic infection. A severe periodontitis is present (Fig. 3.6) causing rapid alveolar bone loss. This early-onset periodontitis in the

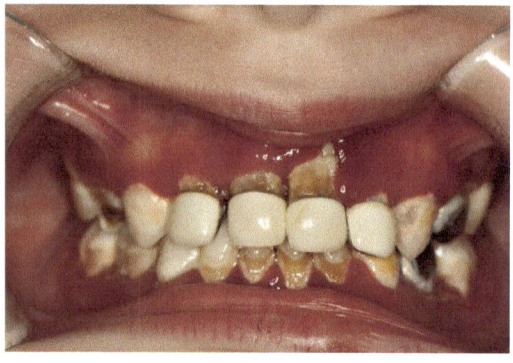

Fig. 3.6 Severe gingivitis and periodontitis associated with leukocyte defect

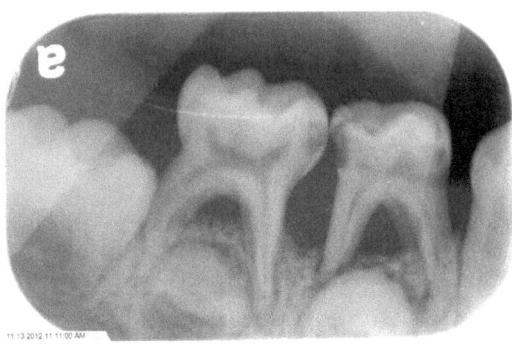

Fig. 3.7 Bone loss associated with the periodontitis seen with leukocyte defect

primary dentition, and the resulting rapid alveolar bone loss (Fig. 3.7) surrounding the primary teeth, is the cause of the early exfoliation of (in some cases) the entire primary dentition [15, 27–29]. A marked gingival inflammation is present around the affected teeth which includes both the primary and permanent dentitions [15, 28] (Table 3.1).

Given the extensive and systemic nature of the course of this disease, the diagnosis may be made by a physician before the patient interacts with a dentist [15, 28]. Dental care includes establishing immaculate oral hygiene, but this is usually not enough to salvage the teeth given the chronic nature of this illness [15, 28]. However, the child represented in Figs. 3.6 and 3.7 had not been diagnosed despite frequent medical visits and it was the oral manifestations and referral by the dentist that lead to the diagnosis.

Neutropenia (Cyclic/Noncyclic)

Neutropenia presents in various forms, each with different etiologies. Neutropenia may be drug induced or idiopathic, acquired or congenital, and cyclic or constant [25]. In children, neutropenia is often the result of the ingestion of medications; however the cyclic form is an autosomal dominant condition (OMIM #162800) [1, 3, 30, 31]. Regardless of the etiology, the pathophysiology is the same. These individuals have a decrease in circulating neutrophils which results in a predisposition for infections including gingivitis, periodontitis, and the premature exfoliation of teeth [25].

Because of the decrease in circulating neutrophils, these children are at increased risk for both opportunistic infections and recurrent infections such as respiratory and skin infections along with otitis media [3]. These children will often have a clinical presentation that also includes fever, malaise, aphthous stomatitis, pharyngitis, regional lymphadenopathy, headache, and conjunctivitis [3].

The dental pathologies reported in children with neutropenia are all associated with an impaired immune system. Severe gingivitis and painful oral ulcerations can be so painful so as to cause difficulty with toothbrushing, eating, and even taking oral medications. If the neutropenia is cyclical in presentation, the gingiva may return to an essentially normal clinical appearance during the time that the neutrophil count returns to normal [1, 3, 30–32].

The recurrent and continued insult to the gingiva and supporting tissue has long-term consequences. Significant loss of supporting bone ultimately occurs. This pronounced loss of alveolar bone results in mobility of both the primary and permanent dentitions [1, 3, 31–33].

Because of the varied etiological factors that can result in neutropenia, onset can occur at any age (if related to the ingestion of a medication), but the onset is shortly after birth or in early childhood for the cyclic neutropenic form [3, 30]. Although it is possible that the first clinical sign noticed could be related to the oral findings, it is much more likely that the diagnosis will be made by a physician prior to presenting to the dental office. Although clinical signs may raise concerns with the physician, the actual diagnosis is made by laboratory studies [25]. Blood analysis and a complete blood count with a differential will demonstrate a depressed neutrophil count (if cyclic, the blood work may need to be done more than once in order to time the test with the transient neutrophil decrease) [31, 32]. Granulocyte colony-stimulating factor is used to treat a variety of neutopenis by stimulating the bone marrow to produce more white blood cells.

The goal of the dental management for these children is to take the measures necessary to prevent the gingival inflammation that ultimately leads to the bone loss, by reducing the amount of dental plaque [33]. Control of this gingival inflammation is attempted by both mechanical and chemotherapeutic measures. Mechanical measures focus on intense preventive/home care which includes scaling and root planing along with extensive oral hygiene and plaque control [30, 32].

Table 3.1 Conditions associated with early exfoliation of primary teeth

Condition	Age of onset	Gingival inflammation	Physical findings	Oral findings	Radiographic findings	Etiology	Specific dental treatment	Add't info
Acrodynia	Variable	Variable	Fever, sweating, anorexia, listlessness, irritability, tachycardia, hypertension	Inflammation and ulceration of mucous membranes	Alveolar bone loss	Exposure to medications with a mercury base in hypersensitive children	Palliative	
Chediak-Higashi syndrome	Variable	Severe	Respiratory and skin infections, strabismus, nystagmus	Early onset and severe destruction of the periodontium	Destruction of alveolar bone	Autosomal recessive inheritance	Palliative	
Singleton-Merten	Variable	Variable	Deformities of the hands and feel, joint subluxation, ruptured ligaments, muscle weakness, short stature, osteoporosis, idiopathic calcification of aortic valve and arch, glaucoma, infertility	Delayed eruption	Alveolar bone loss, delayed root formation, acute root resorption	Autosomal dominant inheritance	Palliative	
Coffin-Lowry syndrome	Birth	Variable	Persistent anterior fontanel, thick hands, extensible joints, generalized hypotonia, sensorineural hearing loss, intellectual disabilities	Furrowed tongue, thick lips, mandibular prognathism, high vaulted palate, microdontia	Alveolar bone loss, no root resorption seen on mobile teeth	X-linked inheritance	Palliative, extraction of mobile symptomatic teeth, aggressive oral hygiene	Hypoplastic cementum present on the roots of affected teeth

Hajdu-Cheney syndrome	In childhood, actual age varies	Yes with bleeding upon probing	Bony dissolution of terminal phalanges of the hands and feet, joint laxity, short stature, scoliosis, kyphosis, elongated skull, small chin, dolichocephalic, coarse hair, thick eyebrows, clubbing of fingers	Gingivitis, periodontitis	Atrophy of alveolar bone, multiple osteolytic lesions, hypoplastic roots, changes in cementum	Autosomal dominant inheritance	Palliative	
Ehlers-Danlos syndrome	Variable	Yes	Hyperextensible skin, hypermobility of the joints of the digits	Enhanced resorption of alveolar bone and root apices resulting in severe alveolar bone loss	Alveolar bone loss, apical root resorption	Autosomal dominant inheritance but multiple subtypes	Palliative, improve oral hygiene as attempt to control loss of attachment	
Papillon-Lefevre syndrome	Approx. the age of eruption of the primary dentition	Yes, hyperemic and edematous gingiva	Hyperkeratosis of the palms of the hands and the soles of the feet	Severe periodontitis with deep periodontal pocketing	Generalized alveolar bone loss	Autosomal recessive inheritance	Aggressive in-office preventive measures (scaling and root planing) with excellent home care and hygiene, use of antibiotics, extraction of hopeless teeth	Can see loss of both dentitions, may consider extraction of all primary teeth in order to allow permanent teeth to erupt into a healthier environment

(continued)

Table 3.1 (continued)

Condition	Age of onset	Gingival inflammation	Physical findings	Oral findings	Radiographic findings	Etiology	Specific dental treatment	Add't info
Cherubism	Between 2 and 4 years of age, mandibular swellings stabilize in size around puberty	Variable	Bilateral mandibular swellings, displacement of ocular globes	Mandibular swellings that can displace primary and permanent teeth	Multilocular radiolucent cystic lesions seen in the ribs or mandible	Autosomal dominant inheritance with highly variable expressivity	Palliative	
Hypophosphatemia	Symptoms evident by 2 years of age	Variable	Short stature, bowed legs	Pulpal exposures with spontaneous abscess	Thin hypomineralized enamel, large pulp chambers, high pulp horns, changes in bony trabeculations, abnormal or absent lamina dura	Variable modes of transmission	Based on patient's presentation; may include pulp therapy with full-coverage crowns along with extraction of abscessed teeth	
Hypothyroidism	Variable	Yes	Increase in circulating thyroid hormone, hyperactivity, emotional disturbances	Accelerated eruption of permanent teeth	Increased bone turnover resulting in bone loss	Increase in circulating thyroid hormone resulting in an increase in the number of bone resorbing cells	Palliative, based on symptoms	
Hypophosphatasia	Variable, but earlier onset associated with increased disease severity and poor prognosis	Minimal inflammation and plaque accumulation	Improper mineralization of bone	Spontaneous tooth loss most often mandibular incisors, enamel hypoplasia, bulbous crowns	Enlarged pulp chambers and root canals, delayed dentin formation	Inherited but multiple forms with varying modes of inheritance	Thorough prevention and oral hygiene	Defective cementum

Prepubertal periodontitis	By 4 years of age	Minimal gingival inflammation seen with localized form; severe acute inflammation with gingival recession seen with generalized form	No specific findings	Possible gingival inflammation with gingival recession	Rapid alveolar bone loss	Seropositive for *Actinobacillus actinomycetemcomitans*	Palliative	
Leukocyte adhesion deficiency	Variable depending on etiology	Marked gingival inflammation	Recurrent fungal and bacterial infections, recurrent skin infections and otitis media. infections of the gastrointestinal tract and mucous membranes	Early-onset periodontitis	Rapid alveolar bone loss	Variable; multiple forms	Establish excellent oral hygiene, but usually not enough to save involved teeth	Affects both primary and permanent dentitions
Neutropenia	Variable	Yes, secondary to the decrease in circulating neutrophils	Predisposition for infections (opportunistic and/or recurrent), fever, malaise, pharyngitis, regional lymphadenopathy, headache, conjunctivitis	Gingivitis, periodontitis, aphthous stomatitis, painful oral ulcers	Loss of alveolar bone support	Various forms; drug induced, idiopathic, cyclic, constant, acquired, congenital	Attempt to prevent gingival inflammation with aggressive plaque control (mechanical and/or chemotherapeutic) but rarely enough to prevent future problems	
Langerhans cell histiocytosis	Usually before 6 years of age	Yes with periodontal pocketing	Vary based on form; fever, skin rashes, otitis media, anemia, lymphadenopathy, hepatosplenomegaly	Alveolar expansion, pain, swelling, halitosis, gingival enlargement, ulcerations, gingival necrosis	Lytic ("punched out") lesions of the bone usually seen in the mandible, teeth appear to be "floating"	Multiple forms with each differing in severity, clinical features, and prognosis	Scaling and root planing, extraction of affected teeth, chlorhexidine	Affects both dentitions

Chemotherapeutic measures can include the use of antibiotics and chlorhexidine [25, 31, 32]. Unfortunately even with vigorous local plaque control measures, many patients are unable to maintain a high enough level of oral hygiene to prevent future disease.

Histiocytosis X/Langerhans Cells

Histiocytosis X (OMIM #602782) is a rare group of disorders that are characterized by a neoplastic or reactive proliferation of histiocytes in various organs or tissues [1, 15, 34, 35]. It occurs most frequently in children (before 6 years of age) or young adults [25, 36]. Some studies report no sex predilection while others report that males are more frequently affected. No racial bias has been reported [25, 34, 36]. Although now referred to as a group as Langerhans cell histiocytosis, this condition does have multiple forms. These forms include Letterer-Siwe disease, Hand-Schuller-Christian, and eosinophilic granuloma [1, 3, 25]. The pathophysiology of each of these all involve Langerhans cells, with a definitive diagnosis being made via biopsy [3, 15, 37].

Each of these forms differs in severity and clinical features [3]. Letterer-Siwe represents the acute and disseminated or fulminating form. This form often affects infants and children who are younger than 3 years of age. Clinically these children suffer from a low-grade fever, erythematous skin rash, thrombocytopenia, anemia, lymphadenopathy, and hepatosplenomegaly along with bony involvement [3, 36]. These bony changes include radiolucent lesions found in the mandible, skull, and long bones [36]. Letterer-Siwe has a very poor prognosis, with most patients dying within a very short period of time [36].

Hand-Schuller-Christian is the disseminated chronic form of Langerhans cell histiocytosis. These individuals also present with frequent fevers and infections, otitis, upper respiratory infections, skin rash, mastoiditis, and lymphadenopathy. Organ involvement includes splenomegaly and hepatomegaly [36].

The mildest and most frequently reported form is eosinophilic granuloma. Even though bony involvement can still occur in any bone including the mandible, clinical features tend to resemble severe juvenile periodontitis [36].

Overall the prognosis for Langerhans cell histiocytosis is poor for the early-onset disseminated form and excellent for the localized mild form [15].

The clinical features associated with Langerhans cell histiocytosis are quite variable, although all forms have some common features [25]. All demonstrate fever, skin rashes, otitis media, anemia, lymphadenopathy, hepatosplenomegaly, and lytic lesions of the bone. All of these features are related to the infiltration by histiocytes of the various end-target organs: skin, bones, liver, and spleen [15, 37].

The reported dental features are a result of the tissue infiltration and the bony lytic "punched out" lesions [35]. Reported oral findings include alveolar expansion with tooth mobility, pain, swelling, halitosis, gingival enlargement, ulcerations, gingival necrosis, premature exfoliation of teeth, periodontal pocketing, and bleeding [1, 3, 15, 25, 34, 36].

The alveolar bone loss is visualized radiographically as discrete destructive radiolucent lesions that give the impression of teeth floating within the alveolar bone [1, 15, 37]. Although these well-defined radiolucencies can occur in many sites (skull, ribs, pelvis, femur, and humerus), the mandible is usually involved with most lesions appearing in the area of the molars (Fig. 3.8) [3, 36].

The treatment varies and is based on the severity of the disease, often requiring radiation therapy and immunosuppressive drugs [25]. Some of the literature discusses periods of observation, but since these lesions are rarely self-limiting, treatment involving surgery, injectable corticosteroids, or low-dose radiation therapy is often necessary [3, 25]. Dental treatment includes scaling and root planing with extraction of affected teeth. Chlorhexidine is also sometimes used [15, 34].

Langerhans cell histiocytosis is a systemic condition that may first be recognized and diagnosed by the dentist. In some cases the oral changes may be the first pathological sign which may lead the patient to seek a dental evaluation [36]. It has been reported in fact that up to 20 % of the cases have their initial tissue infiltration in the oral cavity, usually the mandible [15].

Fig. 3.8 "Floating teeth" as seen on a panoramic radiograph of a patient with Langerhans cell histiocytosis

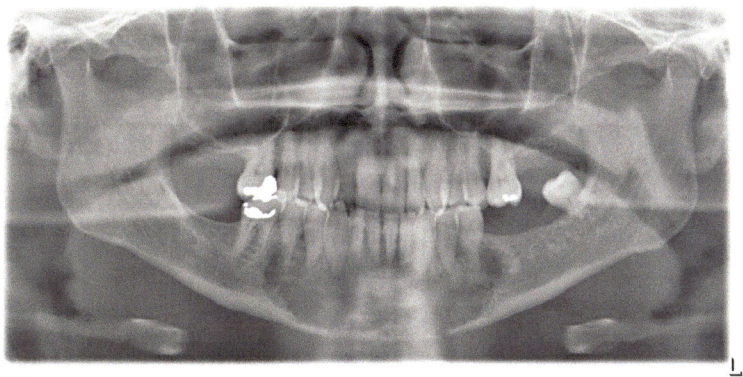

Delayed Eruption of Permanent Teeth

As mentioned earlier, exfoliation of primary teeth and the subsequent eruption of the succedaneous teeth follow a typical pattern and timing. The primary dentition is usually replaced in this process beginning at 6 years of age and is completed at 12 years of age, approximately [38]. However the eruption time can vary considerably.

This variation in eruption time is influenced by many factors. It has been reported that these factors include ethnicity, gender, and race [38, 39]. For example, girls display earlier eruption timing than boys, with an average difference of 4–6 months [39]. It is thought that this is related to the earlier onset of maturity seen in girls [39].

Individual teeth may also display variation within the same dental arch. Lower incisors, for example, demonstrate the least variation in timing of eruption and mandibular second premolars the most [38].

There are also diagnosable conditions that will result in delayed eruption of the permanent dentition (Table 3.2). These conditions can be divided into four general categories. These include gestational, genetic, local, and systemic [39, 40].

Gestational Factors

Preterm Birth
These are related to birth weight and prematurity or preterm, which is a birth weight below 2,500 g or before a gestational age of 37 weeks [39]. Numerous studies have indicated that children born preterm

demonstrate delayed eruption of both primary and permanent dentitions [39]. This delayed eruption is more noticeable in younger children, as the eruption timing seems to catch up as the child ages [39].

Local Factors

Gingival Hyperplasia/Supernumerary Teeth/Ankylosed Teeth/Orofacial Clefts
These factors often result in delayed eruption by acting as a physical obstruction resulting in delayed eruption of the permanent teeth. One such factor is the physical obstruction caused by gingival scar tissue or hyperplasia [39]. This hyperplasia may be the result of pharmacological, hereditary, or hormonal factors [39].

Supernumerary teeth and ankylosis of a primary tooth both have the potential to result in delayed eruption of the permanent dentition, although ankylosis more often results in delayed exfoliation of the primary teeth [39, 40]. Supernumerary teeth, which most often appear in the area of the maxillary incisors (mesiodens), can cause a physical impediment to eruption by causing crowding, displacement, and rotation, resulting in impacted teeth [38, 39].

Delayed eruption has also been reported in children with orofacial clefts [38].

Systemic Factors

Systemic conditions that result in delayed tooth eruption include metabolic, nutritional, and endocrine [39, 40]. Authors have reported that children

Table 3.2 Conditions associated with delayed eruption of permanent teeth

Condition	Age of onset	Physical findings	Oral findings	Etiology	Specific treatment
Premature birth	Birth	Systemic findings based on the degree of prematurity	Delayed eruption of both dentitions	Varies	No condition-specific treatment
Gingival hyperplasia	Varies	Depends on the condition resulting in the hyperplasia	Thickened gingival tissue that covers the teeth and delay eruption	Varies but may be exacerbated by poor oral hygiene	Consultation with a periodontist, gingivectomy, improved oral hygiene, and address underlying etiology
Supernumerary teeth	Varies	Varies, can be the sole finding	Extra teeth will be present clinically or radiographically. These teeth can result in delayed eruption of permanent teeth	Varies	Extraction of supernumerary teeth may be indicated. Monitor growth and development
Ankylosed teeth	Varies	None if not associated with some underlying developmental or medical condition	Teeth appear to be submerged or below the plane of occlusion	Loss of periodontal ligament resulting in direct contact of root surface and alveolar bone	Monitor but extraction may be indicated at some point. Monitor growth and development
Orofacial clefts	Birth	Clefting but severity and location vary	Highly variable	Varies	Refer to pediatric dentist and/or a craniofacial team
Chronic malnutrition	Varies	Varies	Variable but includes delayed eruption of permanent teeth	Insufficient nutritional or caloric intake	Varies, pediatrician or nutritionist will be needed
Hypothyroidism	Varies, could be congenital or acquired	Short stature, short arms and legs, disproportional large head	Smaller dental arches with crowding, large tongue with anterior open bite	Deficiency in circulating thyroid hormone	Careful monitoring of growth and development, may need to refer to an orthodontist
Hypopituitarism	Varies, could be congenital or acquired	Impacts entire body, child appears much younger than chronological age	Delayed eruption of permanent teeth although roots will continue to develop	Decreased function of pituitary gland resulting in decreased secretion or growth hormone	Monitor growth and development, refer to orthodontist and oral surgeon as needed
Apert syndrome	Birth	Syndactyly, polydactyly, exophthalmos, ophthalmoplegia, craniosynostosis	High arched palate, posterior cleft palate, bifid uvula, hypoplastic maxilla, swellings in the maxillary arch associated with the unerupted teeth	Autosomal dominant	Palliative care, monitor growth and development, refer to pediatric dentist and/or craniofacial team

Condition	Age			Inheritance	Management
Gardner syndrome	Birth but age of diagnosis varies	Osteomas, polyps of the gastrointestinal tract, skin and soft tissue tumors, retinal lesion	Supernumerary teeth, malformed teeth, hypercementosis, impacted teeth	Autosomal dominant	Refer to orthodontist to monitor growth and development, refer to oral surgeon for appropriate surgical intervention
Down syndrome	Birth	Characteristic facial appearance includes upwardly sloping eyes with depressed bridge of the nose	Large tongue, small upper face height, dental crowding, significant periodontal disease	Trisomy 21	Aggressive oral hygiene practices, extraction of periodontally hopeless teeth, monitor growth and development
Cleidocranial dysplasia	Birth	Hypoplastic clavicles, open cranial sutures	Hypoplastic midface, dental crowding	Autosomal dominant	Monitor growth and development with referral to orthodontist as appropriate. Extraction of over-retained teeth as needed

who experience chronic malnutrition demonstrate a correlated delayed tooth eruption [39]. Certain endocrine disturbances such as hypothyroidism and hypopituitarism can lead to a delayed eruption [39, 40]. In addition, other disturbances of systemic growth, such as renal problems, can also be linked to delayed eruption [39].

Hypothyroidism

Like all endocrine disorders, hypothyroidism (OMIM #275120) is a disorder that impacts the growth and development of the entire body [39]. This disorder is usually diagnosed at birth by a blood test [40]. Although there are multiple forms of this disorder (congenital versus acquired), the underlying physiological mechanism is similar. Without appropriate treatment, the deficiency in circulating thyroid hormone results in a child who is short in stature with short arms and legs and a disproportionately large head. Obesity is also a common finding [40].

The dental findings in hypothyroidism are also related to the abnormal physical growth. The teeth are normal in size, shape, and number but are crowded in the dental arches because of the smaller jaws [40]. In addition, the tongue appears larger than normal resulting in an anterior open bite [40]. This malocclusion, paired with mouth breathing, results in hyperplasia of the gingiva [40].

Hypopituitarism

As mentioned previously this disorder (OMIM #241540), which is also known as pituitary dwarfism, impacts the child's entire body [39, 40]. Physiologically this decreased function of the pituitary gland results in decreased secretion of growth hormone, which leads to a child who appears much younger than their chronological age. This disorder can also be diagnosed at birth with a blood test [40].

The most significant dental finding associated with hypopituitarism is delayed eruption of the permanent dentition along with delayed exfoliation of the primary teeth. It is interesting to note that the unerupted permanent teeth continue to undergo root development yet often never erupt [40].

Genetic Conditions

There are numerous conditions, some of which were discussed in the Chapter 2, such as Apert and Gardner syndromes, that result in delayed eruption [38–41]. Some of these genetic conditions, along with some of the previously mentioned endocrine disorders, will be discussed in some detail below.

Apert Syndrome

This genetic condition (OMIM #101200) (Fig. 3.9) is characterized by abnormalities in the genes related to fibroblast growth factor receptors. Although the pathological mechanism is unclear, the ultimate result is thickening of the gingiva. Eruption is delayed as the teeth attempt to pass through the thickened gingiva. The swellings associated with these buried teeth of the maxillary arch are a pathognomonic finding [38].

Gardner Syndrome

This rare autosomal dominant condition (OMIM #175100) is known for physical findings in multiple target organs. These physical findings include osteomas, polyps of the gastrointestinal

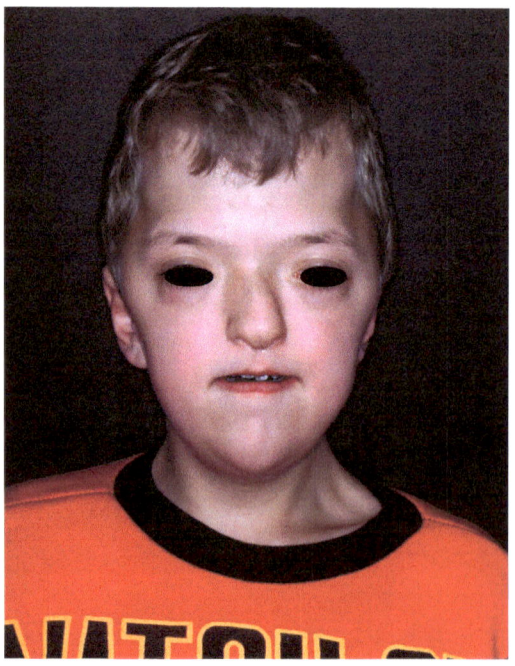

Fig. 3.9 Facial appearance of Apert syndrome

tract, skin and soft tissue tumors, and a lesion of the retina that is pathognomonic for this syndrome [38].

In addition to the above pathologies, dental anomalies are also associated with Gardner syndrome. It has been reported that these dental anomalies are found in up to 75 % of these patients [38]. These anomalies include supernumerary teeth, malformed teeth, fused roots of the molars, hypercementosis, hypodontia, odontomas, and unerupted and impacted teeth. Because of the large number of dental findings, it is possible that the dentist could be the first person to suspect this condition [38].

Down Syndrome

Down syndrome (OMIM #190685) (trisomy 21) is a genetic condition associated with many congenital anomalies including a characteristic facial appearance [40]. These features include upwardly sloping eyes with a bridge of the nose that is depressed more than normal [37]. Many of these children also have malformations of the external part of the ear. More consequential abnormalities are also present such as chronic respiratory infections, impaired immunity, and cardiac problems [40].

Dental findings in children with Down syndrome are numerous and variable. Frequent oral findings include large tongue, small upper face height and midface, gingivitis, significant periodontal disease, and dental crowding [40]. Delayed eruption is also seen along with an abnormal sequence of eruption [40].

Cleidocranial Dysplasia

Cleidocranial dysplasia (OMIM #119600) (CCD) is a rare autosomal dominant condition that is associated with dental anomalies and the characteristic hypoplasia of the clavicle [38, 40, 41]. The prevalence of CCD is estimated to be one per million with sporadic mutations also reported [40, 41].

In addition to the hypoplastic clavicles, other features are common in children with CCD. Some of these include open cranial sutures, small frontal sinuses, hypoplastic midface, and short stature [40, 41].

Dental findings are found in greater than 90 % of affected individuals. Supernumerary teeth along with a shorter maxilla lead to crowding and malocclusions. Delayed eruption of the primary and permanent teeth, along with failure of the primary teeth to exfoliate, is also commonly reported [40, 41].

Conclusion

The early loss of primary teeth and the delayed eruption of the permanent dentition can occur as part of the variation of normal developmental timing. However, as the contents of this chapter indicate, both of these situations can occur as part of the presentation of numerous pathological conditions.

In many of these, treatment interventions do exist so early diagnosis is critical. In addition, knowing the proper course of treatment can have a major impact on the patient's oral health and, by extension, their overall quality of life.

Finally, even though some of these conditions may be best treated by various dental specialists, it is in the patient's best interest if the general dentist can provide early diagnosis along with the appropriate referral in order to help with expediting care.

References

1. Hartsfield JK. Premature exfoliation of teeth in childhood and adolescence. Adv Pediatr. 1994;41:453–70.
2. Sharma G, Whatling R. Case report: premature exfoliation of primary teeth in a 4-year-old child, a diagnostic dilemma. Eur Arch Paediatr Dent. 2011;12(6): 312–7.
3. McDonald RE, Avery DR, Hartsfield JK. Acquired and developmental disturbances of the teeth and associated oral structures. In: McDonald RE, Avery DR, Dean JA, editors. Dentistry for the child and adolescent. 8th ed. St. Louis: Mosby; 2004. p. 103–47.
4. Boraz R. Dental considerations in the treatment of Wiskott-Aldrich syndrome: report of a case. J Dent Child. 1989;56(3):225–7.
5. Armstrong D, Matt M. Auto extraction in an autistic dental patient: a case report. Spec Care Dentist. 1999;19(2):72–4.
6. Bailleul-Forestier I, Monod-Broca J, Benkerrou M, Mora F, Picard B. Generalized periodontitis associated with Chediak-Higashi syndrome. J Periodontol. 2008;79(7):1263–70.

7. Feigenbaum A, Muller C, Yale C, Kleinheinz J, Jezewski P, Kehl HG, MacDougall M, Rutsch F, Hennekam RCM. Singleton-Merten syndrome: an autosomal dominant disorder with variable expression. Am J Med Genet A. 2013;161 A:360–70.

8. Day P, Cole B, Welbury R. Coffin-Lowry syndrome and premature tooth loss: a case report. J Dent Child. 2000;67(2):148–50.

9. Hartsfield JK, Hall BD, Griz AW, Kousseff BG, Salazar JF. Pleiotropy in Coffin-Lowry syndrome: sensorineural hearing deficit and premature tooth loss as early manifestations. Am J Med Genet. 1993;45: 552–7.

10. Norderyd J, Aronsson J. Hypoplastic root cementum and premature loss of primary teeth in Coffin-Lowry syndrome: a case report. Int J Paediatr Dent. 2012;22:154–6.

11. Bazopoulou-Kyrkanidou E, Vrahopoulos TP, Eliades G, Vastardis H, Tosios K, Vrotsos IA. Periodontitis associated with Hajdu-Cheney syndrome. J Periodontol. 2007;78:1831–8.

12. Grant S, Franklin CD, Lund I, Sheffield UK. Acroosteolysis (Hajdu-Cheney) syndrome. Oral Surg Oral Med Oral Pathol Oral Radiol Endod. 1995;80:666–8.

13. Karrer S, Landthaler M, Schmatz G. Ehlers-Danlos type VIII: review of the literature. Clin Oral Invest. 2000;4:66–9.

14. Badauy CM, Gomes SS, Sant'Ana Filho M, Bogo Chies JA. Ehlers-Danlos syndrome (EDS) type IV. Review of the literature. Clin Oral Invest. 2007;11: 183–7.

15. Griffen AC. Periodontal problems in children and adolescents. In: Pinkham JR, Casamassimo PS, McTique DJ, Fields HW, Novak AJ, editors. Pediatric dentistry infancy through adolescence. 4th ed. St. Louis: Elsevier Saunders; 2005. p. 414–22.

16. Patel S, Davidson LE. Papillon-Lefevre syndrome: a report of two cases. Int J Paediatr Dent. 2004;14: 288–94.

17. De Freitas AC, Assed S, da Silva LEA, Silva RAB. Aggressive periodontitis associated with Papillon-Lefevre syndrome: report of a 14-year follow-up. Spec Care Dentist. 2007;27(3):95–100.

18. Canger EM, Celenk P, Devrim I, Yenisey M, Gunhan O. Intraoral findings of Papillon-LeFevre syndrome. J Dent Child. 2008;75:99–103.

19. Prescott T, Redfors M, Fremstad Rustad C, Eiklid KL, Geirdal AO, Storhaug K, Jensen JL. Characteristics of a Norwegian cherubism cohort: molecular genetic findings, oral manifestations and quality of life. Eur J Med Genet. 2013;56:131–7.

20. Fernandes Gomes M, Ferraz de Brito Penna Forte L, Hiraoka CM, Augusto Claro F, Costa Armond M. Clinical and surgical management of an aggressive cherubism treated with autogenous bone graft and calcitonin. ISRN Dent. 2011;2011:340960.

21. Douyere D, Joseph C, Gaucher C, Chaussain C, Courson F. Familial hypophosphatemic vitamin D-resistant rickets- prevention of spontaneous dental abscesses on primary teeth: a case report. Oral Surg Oral Med Oral Pathol Oral Radiol Endod. 2009; 107:525–30.

22. Feitosa DS, Marques MR, Casati MZ, Sallum EA, Nociti FH, de Toledo S. The influence of thyroid hormones on periodontitis-related bone loss and tooth-supporting alveolar bone: a histological study in rats. J Periodontol Res. 2009;44:472–8.

23. Hollis A, Arundel P, High A, Balmer R. Current concepts in hypophosphatasia: case report and literature review. Int J Paediatr Dent. 2013;23:153–9.

24. Mornet E. Hypophosphatasia. Best Pract Clin Rheumatol. 2008;22(1):113–27.

25. Sauk JJ. Defects of the teeth and tooth-bearing structures. In: Braham RL, Morris ME, editors. Textbook of pediatric dentistry. 2nd ed. Baltimore: Williams and Wilkins: 1985. pp. 72–104.

26. Whyte MP, Greenberg CR, Salman NJ, Bober MB, McAlister WH, et al. Enzyme-replacement therapy in life-threatening hypophosphatasia. N Engl J Med. 2012;366(10):904–13.

27. Majorana A, Notarangelo LD, Savoldi E, Gastaldi G, Lozada-Nur F. Leukocyte adhesion deficiency in a child with severe oral involvement. Oral Surg Oral Med Oral Pathol Oral Radiol Endod. 1999;87:691–4.

28. Dababneh R, Al-wahadneh AM, Hamadneh S, Khouri A, Bissada NF. Periodontal manifestations of leukocyte adhesion deficiency type I. J Periodontal. 2008;79:764–8.

29. Nagendran J, Anandakrishna L, Prakash C, Gaviappa D, Ganesh D. Leukocyte adhesion deficiency: a case report and review. J Dent Child. 2012;79(2):105–10.

30. Da Fonseca MA, Fontes F. Early tooth loss due to cyclic neutropenia: long-term follow-up of one patient. Spec Care Dent. 2000;20(5):187–90.

31. Hakki SS, Aprikyan AAG, Yildirum S, Aydinbelge M, Gokalp A, Ucar C, Gurman S, Koseoglu V, Ataaglu T, Somerman MJ. Periodontal status in two siblings with severe congenital neutropenia: diagnosis and mutational analysis of the cases. J Periodontol. 2005;76:837–44.

32. Zaromb A, Chamberlain D, Schoor R, Almas K, Blei F. Periodontitis as a manifestation of chronic benign neutropenia. J Periodontol. 2006;77:1921–6.

33. Antonio AG, da Costa Alcantoro PC, Ramos MEB, de Souza IPR. The importance of dental care for a child with severe congenital neutropenia: a case report. Spec Care Dentist. 2010;30(6):261–5.

34. Torrungruang K, Sittisomwong S, Rojansomith K, Asvanit P, Korkong W, Vipismak V. Langerhans' cell histiocytosis in a 5-year-old girl: evidence of periodontal pathogens. J Periodontol. 2006;77:728–33.

35. Ladisch S. Langerhans cell histiocytosis. Curr Opin Hematol. 1998;5:54–8.

36. Rapp GE, Motta ACE. A clinical case of Langerhans' cell histiocytosis. Braz Dent J. 2000;11(1):59–66.

37. Aldred MJ, Crawford PJM, Day A, Dallimore N. Precocious tooth eruption and loss in Letterer-Siwe disease. Br Dent J. 1988;165(10):367–70.

38. Klein OD, Oberoi S, Huysseune A, Hovorakova M, Peterka M, Peterkova R. Developmental disorders of the dentition: an update. Am J Med Genet. 2013;163:318–32.

39. Peedikayil FC. Delayed tooth eruption. J Dent. 2011;1(4):81–6.

40. McDonald RE, Avery DR, Hartsfield JK. Eruption of the teeth: local, systemic, and congenital factors that influence the process. In: McDonald RE, Avery DR, Dean JA, editors. Dentistry for the child and adolescent. 8th ed. St. Louis: Mosby; 2004. p. 174–202.

41. Cooper SC, Flaitz CM, Johnston DA, Lee B, Hecht JT. A natural history of cleidocranial dysplasia. Am J Med Genet. 2001;104:1–6.

Treatment of Nonsyndromic Anomalies of Tooth Number

4

Lyndon F. Cooper

Abstract

Nonsyndromic tooth agenesis represents a common odontogenic condition that should be managed by a multidisciplinary specialty team. The genetic basis for agenesis of teeth reflects the key transcriptional events involved in mesenchymal-epithelial interactions during tooth formation. Mutations of genes including *PAX9*, *MSX1*, *AXIN2*, and *EDA* are implicated. Clinicians should be aware of familial history of tooth agenesis. Treatment may involve orthodontists and prosthodontists early in the management of these individuals. In all cases, the establishment of oral health, stable occlusion, and establishment of a conceptual framework for treatment resulting in efficient tooth replacement and aesthetic outcomes should be considered in the mixed dentition phase. Definitive tooth replacement using conventional or implant prostheses should be reserved for individuals with complete facial growth and maturation.

Introduction

Beyond caries and trauma, a third common cause of a missing tooth or teeth requiring treatment is the spectrum of developmental anomalies that result in enamel or dentin hypoplasia, tooth dysplasia, or tooth agenesis [23]. While several of these developmental tooth anomalies of genetic basis are part of well-described syndromes, other variations in the number of teeth result from nonsyndromic and unique (not inherited) disruption in the genetically encoded program and molecular pathways necessary for tooth development. On occasion, hypodontia can be attributable to environmental factors that disrupt this developmental program such as infection (e.g., rubella), trauma, chemo- or radiotherapy, or disturbances in jaw innervations [25]. While the topic of syndromic tooth agenesis is the focus of the accompanying chapter by Dr. Clark Stanford (see Chap. 5), the dual purpose of this report is to review the molecular basis for nonsyndromic tooth agenesis and to illustrate the contemporary clinical management of the varied clinical conditions representing this spectrum of genetically based disorders.

L.F. Cooper, DDS, PhD
Department of Prosthodontics,
University of North Carolina at Chapel Hill,
Chapel Hill, NC, USA
e-mail: Lyndon_Cooper@unc.edu

The Spectrum of Nonsyndromic Selective Tooth Agenesis

Selective tooth agenesis (STHAG) has been proposed as a term to describe the full spectrum of disorders of tooth number [9]. Included within this term are the classically defined terms, hypodontia, oligodontia, and anodontia (Table 4.1).

When considering the nonsyndromic forms of selective tooth agenesis, agenesis is reported to affect any of the permanent teeth with varying prevalence that is variable among different populations and races [16]. The most commonly missing teeth include third molars (excluded from definitions of oligodontia and hypodontia), mandibular second premolars, and lateral incisors. Current estimations suggest that hypodontias affect approximately 7–8 % of the population and oligodontias are displayed by less than 0.5 % of the population [15]. Reports of anodontia are extremely rare.

Nonsyndromic selective tooth agenesis represents the most common form of congenital tooth agenesis. It has been classified as either sporadic or familial and is inherited in autosomal dominant, autosomal recessive, or X-linked modes [5]. The observed clinical diversity underscores the considerable variation in both penetrance and expression. Nonsyndromic selective tooth agenesis commonly affects the secondary dentition; rarely is it observed in the primary dentition (Fig. 4.1). This finding has many implications for clinical management. Principally, the management begins with evaluation and treatment of the primary or mixed dentition while considering the needs of the adolescent and young adult patient. When man-

Table 4.1 Classifications of selective tooth agenesis

Inheritance	Magnitude	Definition
Syndromic	Hypodontia	Less than six teeth absent
Nonsyndromic	Oligodontia	Six or more teeth absent
	Anodontia	All permanent (and/or deciduous) teeth absent

aging patients with developmentally missing teeth, it is critical to have in mind both the short-term and long-term goals as you set forth on a treatment trajectory. The clinician should always have a vision for what future treatment may be necessary to achieve those goals.

The Molecular Basis of Nonsyndromic Selective Tooth Agenesis

Agenesis of one or more teeth is a result of errors in the earliest processes of development. The first morphological cues are found in the thickening of the oral epithelium to form to dental lamina, and the inductive, tooth-forming potential arises from the dental ectoderm. The next steps, now directed by the dental mesenchyme, lead to the formation of the epithelial bud, and shortly thereafter the enamel knot is formed and reacquires directed control of morphogenesis. Subsequently, the cap stage is recognized and progresses by mesenchymal-epithelial interactions to the bell stage in which fully committed ameloblastic cells and odontoblastic cells surrounding the dental papilla follow a complex genetic program leading to complete tooth development [17, 26]. The mesenchymal cells differentiate into odontoblasts. The opposing epithelial cells differentiate into ameloblasts.

The morphologic description of tooth development (proceeding from dental lamina, to bud, to cap, to bell stages) is temporally associated with a pattern of regulated gene expression. Prominent among these events is the expression of regulatory molecules that play key roles in differentiation and development. Evidence of the roles that specific genes play in the location, size, shape, and number of teeth has come from genetic investigations conducted in mice [21, 22]. Many others have recently reviewed the remarkable molecular events that direct the formation of teeth [27]. Over 300 genes, many of which encode growth factors, transcription factors, or receptors, have been identified to contribute in this process

Fig. 4.1 Diversity of nonsyndromic tooth agenesis represented in young adults. (**a**) Panoramic radiograph reveals absence of the right maxillary lateral incisor tooth and a peg malformation of the maxillary left lateral incisor. (**b**) More extensive agenesis with only 14 permanent teeth present. Note that the management has involved the retention of mandibular lateral incisors and canine teeth as well as molars. (**c**) Extensive tooth agenesis revealing the presence of 12 permanent teeth with malformation

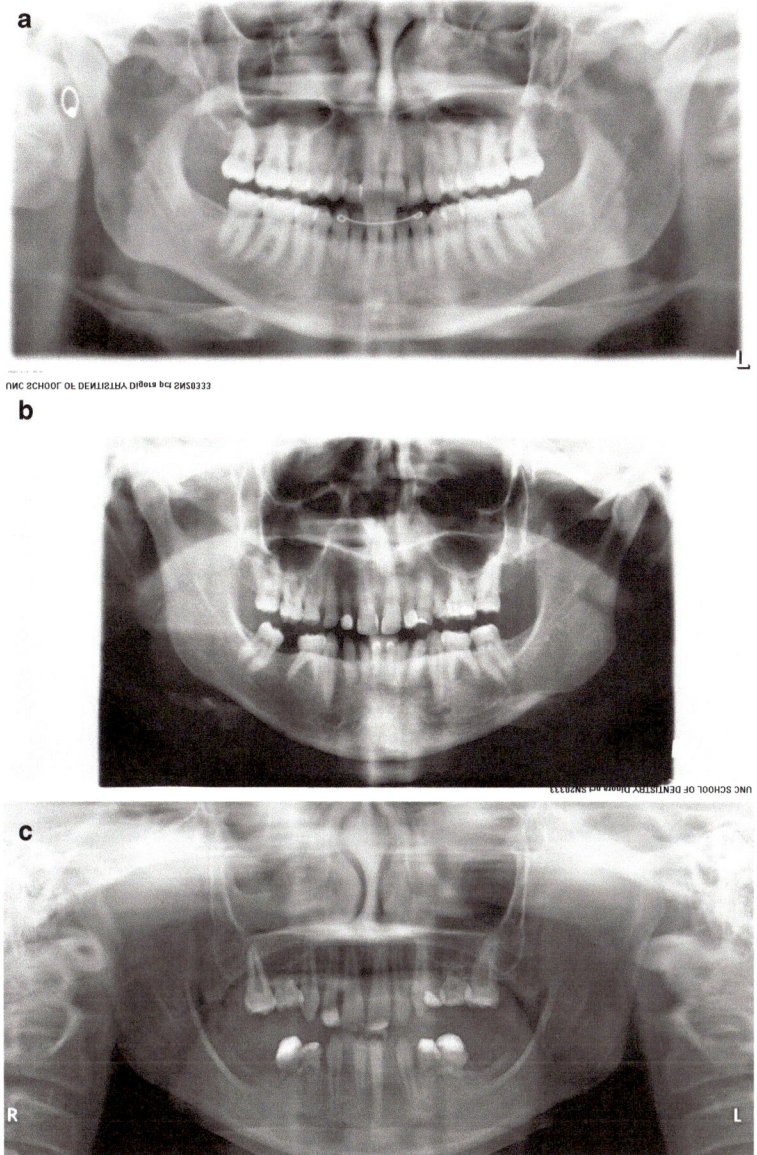

[22]. By way of a brief summary, several specific known genetic alterations have been associated with nonsyndromic selective tooth agenesis (Table 4.2).

Development is fundamentally regulated by homeobox-encoding genes that serve as master transcriptional regulators or genes that produce proteins that orchestrate the expression of other genes and their protein products. Included are *MSX1* and *MSX2*. In tooth development, *MSX1* gene expression

contributes to early stages of tooth development. The disruption of *Msx1* in mice causes developmental arrest of incisor and molar teeth [7]. Deletion, frameshift, and nonsense mutations of *MSX1* (OMIM #106600 – STHAG1) in humans are associated with inherited forms of nonsyndromic and syndromic forms (Witkop syndrome – OMIM #189500) of tooth agenesis [19, 24].

PAX9 gene mutations are also associated with nonsyndromic selective tooth agenesis (OMIM

Table 4.2 Gene mutations associated with nonsyndromic selective tooth agenesis

Gene	Phenotype	Inheritance
MSX1	Hypodontia	Autosomal dominant
	Oligodontia	Autosomal recessive
PAX9	Molar hypodontia	Autosomal dominant
	Oligodontia	
AXIN2	Incisor agenesis	Autosomal dominant
EDA	Hypodontia	X-linked recessive
LTBP3	Oligodontia	Autosomal recessive
WNT10A	Oligodontia	Autosomal dominant

Genes associated with nonsyndromic tooth agenesis can also be associated with syndromes, making it critical to thoroughly evaluate each case and derive a correct diagnosis

#604625 – STHAG3). PAX9 is another homeodomain protein that directly activates the *MSX1* gene. A central and early regulatory role in tooth development is evidenced in *Pax9* homozygous deficient mice that lack all teeth for which development is arrested in the bud stage. Severe hypodontia in humans can be a result of *PAX9* haploinsufficiency (one gene allele produces no functional protein, while the other *PAX9* allele produces normal protein) [10] or different frameshift, deletion, missense, or nonsense mutations in the *PAX9* gene.

The WNT gene family of morphogens is broadly active in human development, especially where mesenchymal-epithelial interactions are prominent such as the process exemplified by tooth development. Inhibition of the WNT pathway causes arrest of tooth development prior to the bud stage [1]. Wnt protein-induced signaling culminates in transcriptional regulation involving β-catenin. AXIN2 is a Wnt-signaling pathway protein that regulates β-catenin activity. Mutations of *AXIN2* were found among individuals with different tooth agenesis patterns, and these individuals were identified to have an increased risk of colon cancer. Therefore individuals with *AXIN2* mutations are considered as having oligodontia-colorectal cancer syndrome (OMIM #608615). Interestingly, Gardner syndrome (OMIM # 175100) is associated with supernumerary teeth and increased risk of colon cancer and results from mutations in the APC gene

which also is in the β-catenin pathway. In a recent study, mutations in the *WNT10A* gene accounted for almost a third of selective tooth agenesis cases (STHAG4 – OMIM #150400) [3]. *WNT10A* mutations also are associated with syndrome-associated missing teeth (odontoonychodermal dysplasia, OMIM # 257980, and Schopf-Schulz-Passarge syndrome, OMIM #224750). Diverse mutations of inherited and spontaneous nature have been identified and lead to varying degrees of oligodontia and hypodontia [26]. The association of missing teeth with very diverse syndromes, some of which have significant other potential occult manifestations such as colon cancer risk, amplifies the need for obtaining a correct diagnosis of the etiology in all cases of selective tooth agenesis.

The more common forms of ectodermal dysplasias and related tooth agenesis conditions are due to mutations of the ligands, receptors, and signaling molecules along a tumor necrosis factor-related pathway represented by EDA (the ligand), EDAR (the receptor), EDARADD (signaling adaptor), the IKK gamma (NEMO) kinase, and WNT10A [8, 14]. However, a nonsyndromic X-linked mutation was associated with an *EDA* gene mutation expressed as the congenital absence of maxillary and mandibular central incisors, lateral incisors, and canines [11].

Other genes may be implicated in nonsyndromic selective tooth agenesis. Recently, *LTBP3* (latent TGF-β binding protein 3) mutation was identified as responsible for an autosomal recessive form of familial oligodontia. Because genetic evaluation of individuals with oligodontia or hypodontia has not yet become fully integrated in the management of these individuals, it is likely that – with further screening – other genes and mutations will be identified as responsible for the spontaneous and familial expression of nonsyndromic selective tooth agenesis.

Clinical Diagnosis and Genetic Evaluations

The phenotypic expression of nonsyndromic tooth agenesis is varied and latent. A clinical evaluation of the primary dentition may reveal subtle or no clues to the developmental changes in the permanent dentition. An early clue may be retention of primary teeth and alterations in lateral incisor morphology. Nonsyndromic tooth agenesis may be inherited, and a dental history should include inquiry regarding family member dental status. When developmentally missing teeth are suspected then radiographic evaluation of the mixed dentition will ultimately reveal the absence of the affected teeth.

Once the developmental absence of permanent teeth is revealed, early collaboration among dental specialists is essential to develop short-term and long-term treatment objectives and goals. As the severity of tooth agenesis increases, attendant alterations in alveolar bone volume ultimately influencing maxillary and mandibular dimension can occur. A proper diagnosis must account for more global, skeletal changes associated with oligodontias.

Proper management of nonsyndromic tooth agenesis focuses on preserving teeth and the replacement of missing teeth for aesthetic, functional, and social reasons. The prevention of caries and periodontal diseases is paramount. Thus, a proper diagnosis must include a caries risk assessment and the subsequent management of this risk. The preservation of teeth and their possible orthodontic movement and strategic utilization are vitally important in the management of nonsyndromic tooth agenesis.

Interdisciplinary Treatment Plans

Management of individuals with nonsyndromic selective tooth agenesis reflects its impact on the dentition and the specific clinical phenotype. Because the deciduous teeth are less commonly affected by nonsyndromic tooth agenesis, concern and related management typically begins with the mixed dentition. In most cases, size discrepancies between retained deciduous teeth and the positionally related permanent teeth are significant. To avoid restorative complications and aesthetic limitations, coordination between pediatric, orthodontic, and prosthodontic specialists should be initiated early in the process of management. This will allow management of the patient's aesthetic and functional concerns while planning for the definitive future treatment plan. Depending on the extent of tooth agenesis, there may be more general concerns. The management of one or two single missing teeth requires consideration of local factors related to the retention of the primary tooth, primary tooth removal, and space maintenance, as well as general concerns related to caries prevention and orthodontic tooth movement. When the expressed mutation results in a growing number of missing teeth, additional concerns regarding possible malocclusion, alveolar bone growth, and related craniofacial growth and development (in the absence of any syndrome) become important.

Recommended is an early evaluation of the patient and consultation by the pediatric, orthodontic, and prosthodontic specialist. In the mixed dentition phase, the prosthodontist should offer a possible therapeutic goal(s) for missing tooth replacement. Depending on patient and parent concerns, finances, and oral and systemic health factors, the solutions offered can involve orthodontic solutions, simple removable prostheses, tooth-supported fixed prosthodontic solutions, and, more commonly today, dental implant-supported fixed prosthodontic solutions.

The primary prosthodontic concerns are to (1) preserve all teeth and maintain ideal periodontal health during the transition period from a mixed dentition to a permanent dentition, (2) maintain ideal dental midline and occlusal plane orientations throughout treatment, and (3) maximize (not reduce) alveolar dimensions to create more ideal tooth positions and facial aesthetics for the final prosthetic plan in adulthood. To achieve these goals, the pediatric dentist must optimize caries control, especially during orthodontic intervention. The orthodontist must provide realistic estimations of the extent to which teeth may be moved to maintain natural tooth dimensions of edentulous spaces and, in cases of oligodontias, how the reductions in alveolar dimension (both vertically and horizontally) may be influenced by orthodontics to reach or approximate an acceptable lower third facial height and to assist in providing acceptable maxillomandibular relationships. At this early period of intervention,

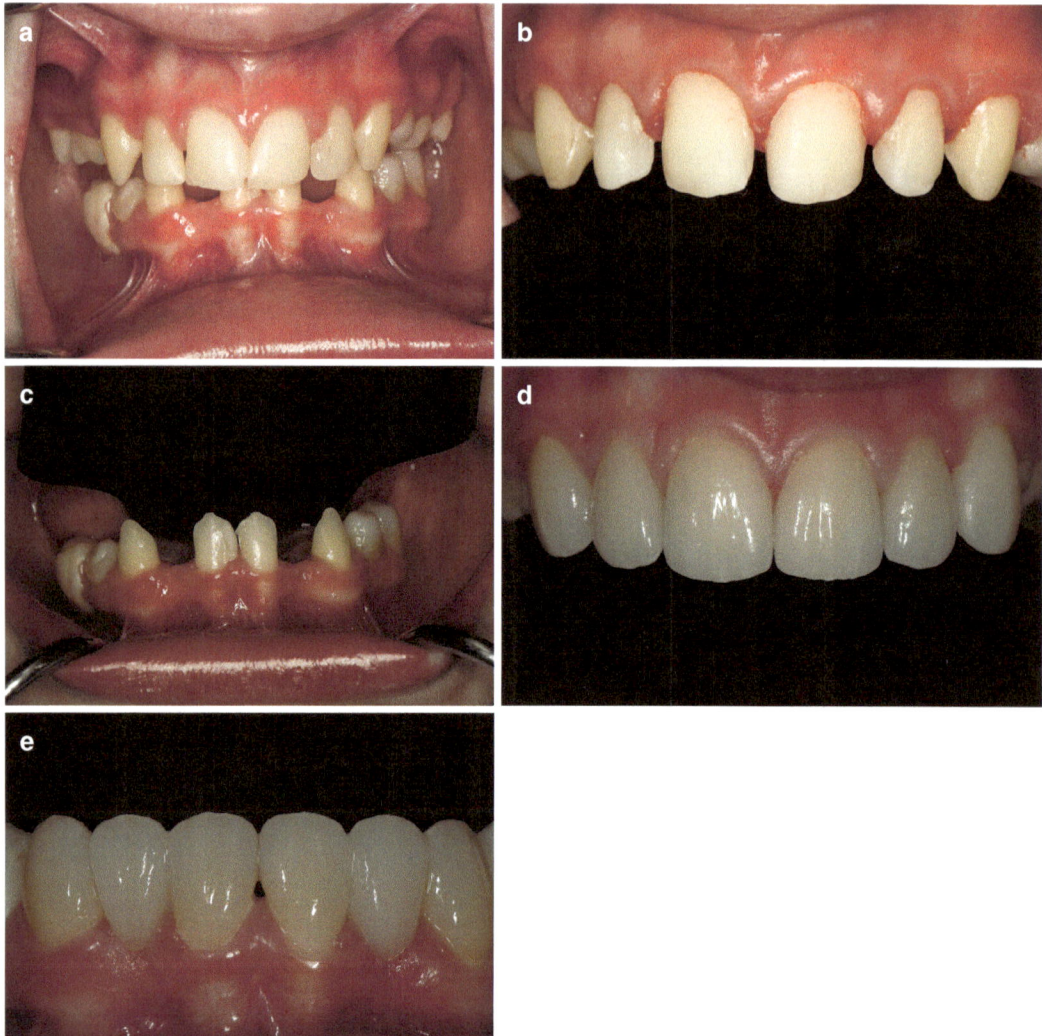

Fig. 4.2 (**a**) Facial intraoral photograph of a 14-year-old female patient with nonsyndromic tooth agenesis represented in Fig. 4.1c. Note the initial attempt to close all spaces of maxillary anterior teeth. (**b**) Intraoral photograph of maxillary anterior tooth following preparation for ceramic veneers at 18 years of age. The tooth spacing was refined by orthodontics prior to tooth preparation. (**c**) Intraoral photograph of mandibular anterior teeth following orthodontic movement to permit placement of all-ceramic bonded restorations replacing the lateral incisors. (**d**) Intraoral facial photograph of the maxillary anterior teeth following restoration using ceramic veneers. (**e**) Intraoral facial photograph of the mandibular anterior teeth following restoration using bonded all-ceramic fixed dental prostheses

the prosthodontist should help to guide treatment toward a clearly elucidated and invariant final therapeutic goal and provide interim solutions for aesthetic and phonetic (anterior) tooth replacement in the mixed dentition. An example of this early interaction, its outcome in the permanent dentition, and the eventual restoration is illustrated in Fig. 4.2.

Interim Treatment Options

Throughout treatment, the missing teeth and spacing created for definitive restorations will require management. It is likely that during orthodontic intervention, prosthetic teeth will be retained on orthodontic wires and on removable orthodontic appliances. However, in a retention phase of treatment, when the patient is too young

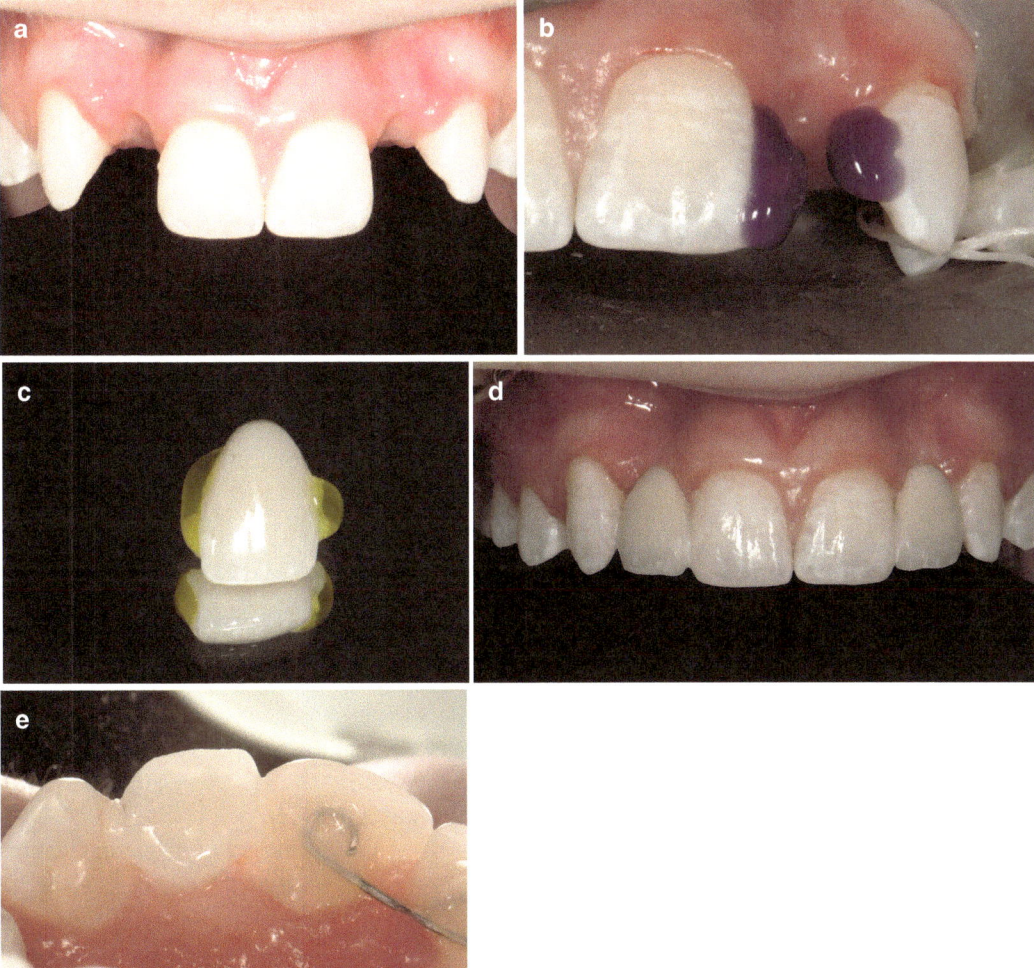

Fig. 4.3 Presentation of a 15 year old female patient with lateral incisor agenesis. Note the residual alveolar ridge resorption is severe, and implant therapy will require bone augmentation at a later date. (**a**) Bonded pontic strategy for long-term provisionalization was selected. (**b**) Etching of the adjacent proximal enamel surfaces, (**c**) hydrofluoric acid etching of the interproximal surfaces of the ceramic (e max) pontic, (**d**) lingual view of the bonded pontic (note the absence of extensive lingual wings of this provisional design), and (**e**) intraoral facial photograph of the bonded pontics replacing maxillary right and left lateral incisors. The intent of this treatment is to provide a fixed solution for provisionalization for 3–5 years

for conventional fixed prosthodontic treatment (due to relatively large pulp chambers precluding tooth preparation or to facial growth concerns), dental implant therapy concerns related to both alveolar and facial growth concerns, as well as practical or financial reasons, removable partial prostheses or bonded pontics [12] may be provided (Fig. 4.3).

Lifelong Care and Dental Implant Therapy for Oligodontias and Hypodontias

The expression of genes with mutations leading to nonsyndromic tooth agenesis may influence a single tooth. Most commonly, this is observed in adulthood as the single missing lateral incisor (or

Table 4.3 Tooth replacement for nonsyndromic selective tooth agenesis

Method	Advantages	Disadvantages
Removable partial denture	Reversible	Removable (unstable, loss)
	Simple repair	Relative lower aesthetics
	Lower cost	Associated candidiasis
	No or little tooth preparation	Risk of fracture
Bonded pontic	Reversible, yet fixed	Technique sensitive
	Lower cost	Impedes interproximal hygiene
	Little tooth preparation	Untimely debonding
	Higher aesthetic potential	
Conventional FDP	Fixed	Risk of pulpal necrosis
	Higher aesthetic potential	Risk of recurrent caries
	Durability	Technique sensitive
		Cost
Dental implant	Fixed	Risk of relative tooth extrusion
	Higher aesthetic potential	Risk of periimplantitis
	Durability	Component complications
	No tooth preparation	May involve multiple surgical interventions
		Cost

Note that all of these alternatives may involve preprosthetic orthodontic and/or periodontal interventions

premolar). Orthodontists most commonly manage these unilateral situations symmetrically with the result being a single missing lateral incisor or premolar. On occasion, premolar extractions provide resolution without need for prosthetic intervention.

A single tooth may be replaced using removable prostheses, conventional fixed dental prostheses, resin-bonded prostheses, or dental implants. Most recently, both clinical data regarding success of prostheses [28] and cost utility data [20] comparing implants and teeth indicate that there may be some benefit to the lifetime utilization of a carefully placed and restored dental implant. Patients who receive dental implants for single-tooth replacement display notable increases in oral health-related quality of life [29], and this is true for tooth agenesis patients [6]. While Implants should be reserved for individuals who have completed facial growth (typically beyond teenage years and approaching early 20s), a long-term potential complication of dental implant placement is relative implant tooth intrusion over time [2]. It must be acknowledged that this problem is not restricted to young patients [4], but it is a concern, and any treatment option must be provided with complete informed consent to the consenting parent and/or patient to educate the patient and parent or guardian fully about the risks and benefits of the alternative treatments (Table 4.3).

Among the advantages of single-implant restorations to replace a single missing tooth are (1) preservation of adjacent tooth structure and reduced risk of adjacent tooth failure, (2) maintenance of alveolar bone following implant restoration and function, and (3) opportunity for ideal aesthetics and function when all procedures are performed well. Some of the key disadvantages in selection of the single-implant restoration are (1) perceived high initial cost and (2) risk of early implant failure (addressed by replacement), risk of late failure due to periimplantitis, and relative implant crown intrusion. Taken together, when financial matters are manageable, the dental implant solution provided by experienced clinical specialists offers many more advantages than disadvantages to the young adult seeking a lifetime of service in replacement of the missing tooth (Fig. 4.4).

Hypodontias involving several missing teeth frequently include bilaterally absent maxillary lateral incisors. Other teeth are less frequently bilaterally absent (e.g., Fig. 4.4). While canine

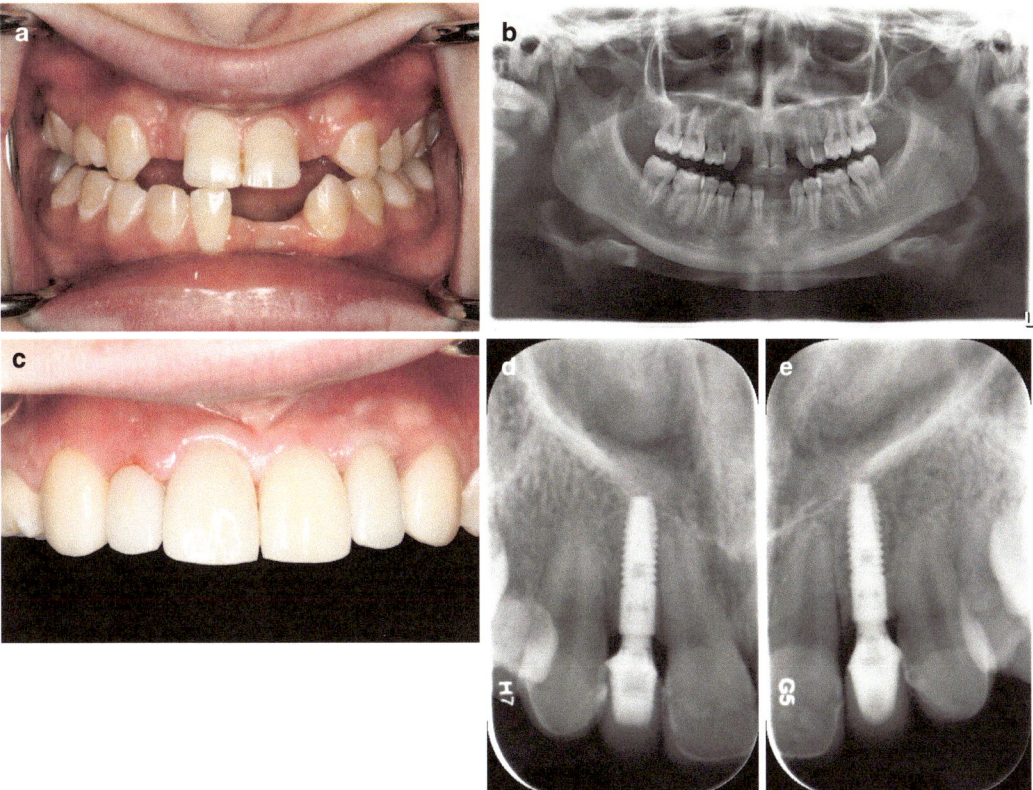

Fig. 4.4 (**a**) Agenesis involves many teeth often with asymmetrical presentation (maxillary right premolar and mandible). (**b**) Pretreatment panoramic radiograph revealing the result of multispecialty treatment involving caries prevention and orthodontics coordinated with the prosthetic plant to replace missing incisors using dental implants. (**c**) The resulting maxillary tooth replacement using all-ceramic crowns and single-tooth implants for each missing lateral incisor tooth. (**d**, **e**) Posttreatment radiographs of the right and left maxillary incisor implants, abutments, and crowns

substitution that typically involves orthodontic position and reshaping canines to resemble the lateral incisor is regarded as one alternative treatment, resin-bonded prostheses or dental implants represent aesthetic alternatives. The key advantages to the canine substitution approach are the reduction or absence of economic, practical, and biologic costs and risk associated with prosthetic and implant interventions [13]. The difficulties encountered using this approach are aesthetic and include (a) tooth size discrepancies (large canines vs. smaller lateral incisors), (b) tooth color discrepancies (darker canine shade, high chroma), (c) aberrant gingival morphology, and, in a related manner, (d) relatively "short" premolar teeth in the canine positions. Constriction of the maxillary arch could, especially in cases of maxillary insufficiency, contribute further to reduced lower face dimension. Unilateral canine substitutions are further exacerbated in efforts to achieve symmetry that drives aesthetic excellence.

Hypodontias involving two or more teeth do occasionally involve adjacent teeth. These conditions create unique problems for eventual restoration by the prosthodontist. For the case of conventional prostheses using teeth as abutments, a longer-span fixed dental prosthesis is required and may involve additional abutment teeth. When the complexity (number of teeth) of a fixed dental prosthesis is increased, the complication rate increases and the prosthesis longevity is reduced.

Alternatively, when selecting dental implants to replace two adjacent teeth, there are aesthetic limitations related to the interproximal tissue dimensions between two implants. It is presently not possible to fully reconstruct the interproximal

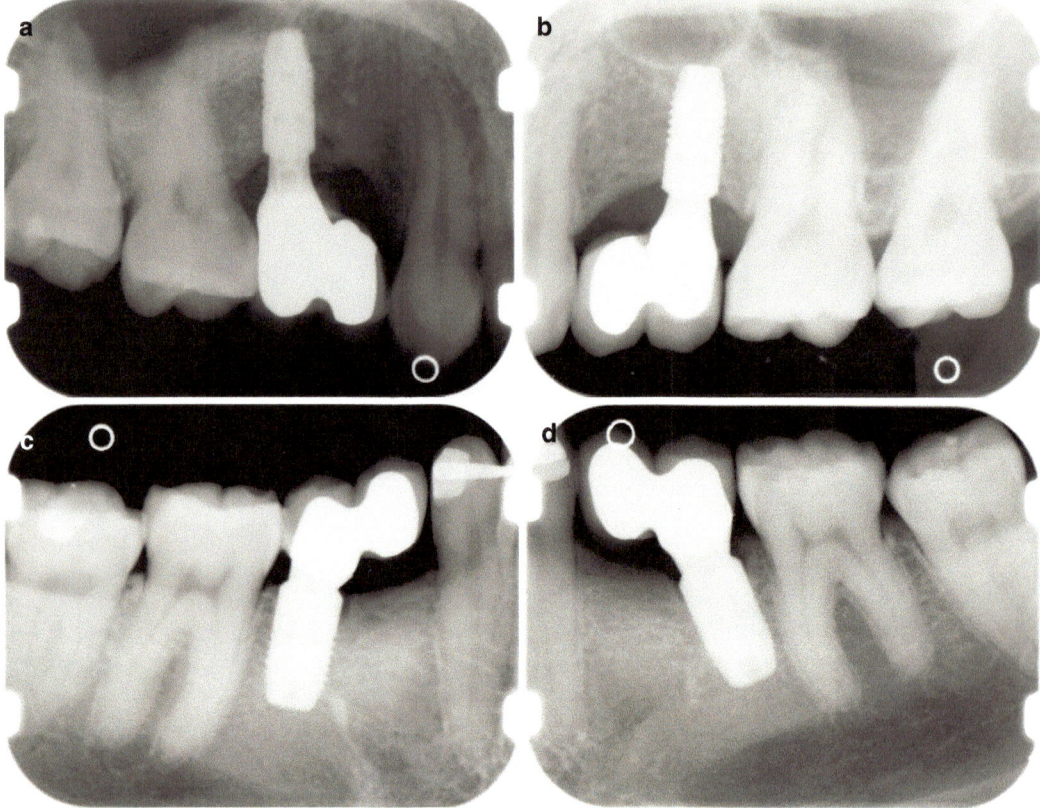

Fig. 4.5 Complete bicuspid agenesis was addressed orthodontically by maintenance of spacing for first and second bicuspids. Here the resulting treatment involved the use of only one implant per quadrant and the restoration using mesial cantilever fixed dental prostheses. Implants replacing teeth maxillary right (**a**), maxillary left (**b**), mandibular right (**c**), and mandibular left (**d**) are shown in the postoperative radiographs

tissues between two dental implants. While one solution is to utilize a single implant, there exists little data to provide guidance here when considering the promise of lifelong function for a young patient. For example, it is known that a cantilever prosthesis for dental implants is associated with lower implant survival and higher prosthetic complications [18]. With careful application of sufficiently large implant components and smaller cantilevers oriented in a mesial position relative to the implant abutment, it may be possible to offer simple, single-implant solutions for two adjacent missing teeth. Properly informing the patient regarding the additional incremental risks of complications and carefully training the patient to perform oral hygiene around the implant and beneath the pontic are essential aspects of managing these patients (Fig. 4.5).

A third approach to solving this problem in a proactive manner is to coordinate treatment with the orthodontist to "split" the adjacent missing tooth spaces by orthodontic movement of the next adjacent tooth into this space. It is acknowledged that this approach will create two bound edentulous spaces into which two dental implants must be placed and there are attendant additional costs. However, in some circumstances, this approach may offer more ideal management of a difficult aesthetic or functional scenario.

Nonsyndromic hypodontias are represented by a wide array of missing tooth positions and combinations that are often bilateral but not uncommonly unilaterally distributed (Figs. 4.1a and 4.4b). When multiple teeth are absent, the primary goal of the dental specialist team is to preserve as many teeth as possible. Not unrecognized is that

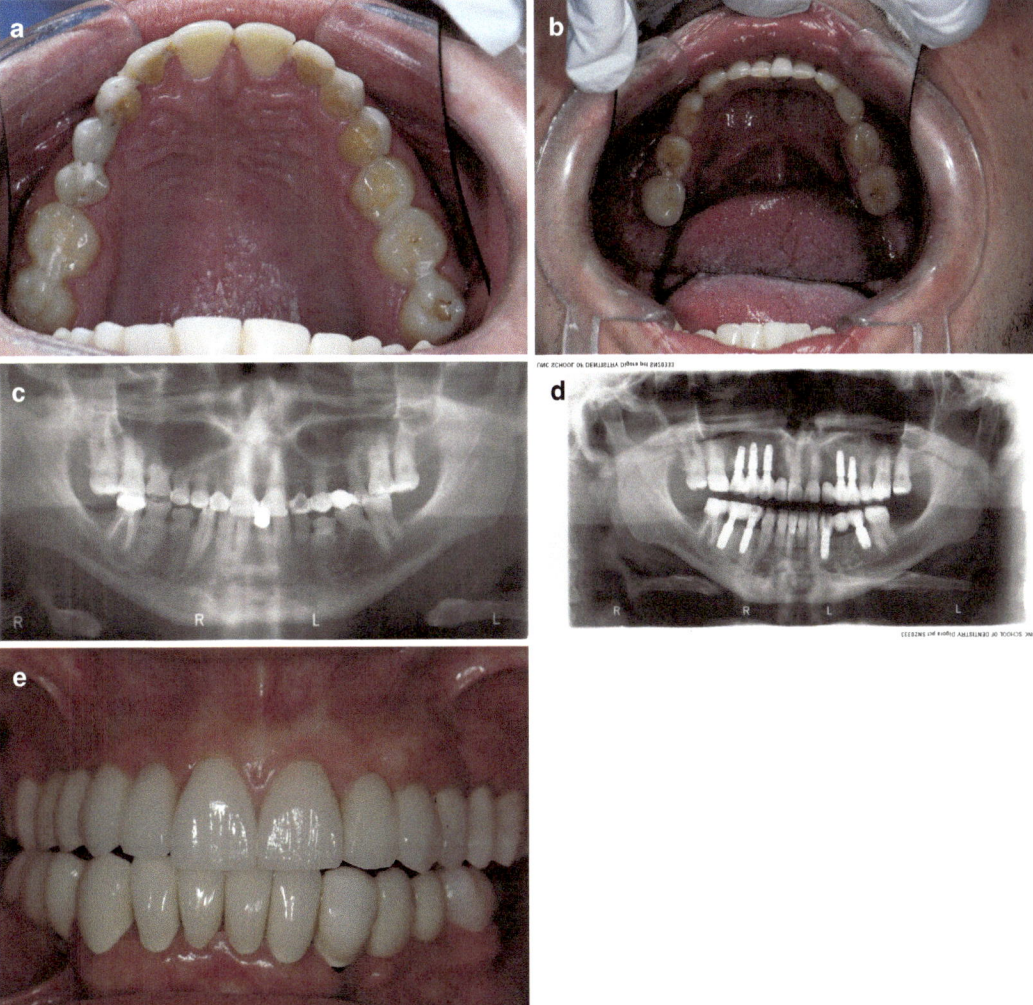

Fig. 4.6 Treatment of extensive nonsyndromic tooth agenesis. (**a**) Preprosthetic treatment occlusal photograph reveals extensive management of existing teeth using composite materials and a resin-bonded prosthesis. (**b**) Interproximal and occlusal contacts have been managed over time using composite restorations of the mandibular retained deciduous teeth. (**c**) Preprosthetic treatment panoramic radiograph reveals the retention of ten deciduous teeth and their restoration in management of adolescent needs for aesthetics. At this time the patient was over 20 years old and prepared to undergo comprehensive prosthodontic therapy. (**d**) Post-prosthetic treatment panoramic radiograph demonstrates the replacement of deciduous teeth and missing permanent teeth using dental implants. Note mesial cantilevers are used in replacement of the lateral incisor teeth. (**e**) Intraoral facial photograph of the patient in protrusive position at 1-year recall appointment

the permanent teeth may be morphologically unique and frequently smaller. These smaller teeth should be preserved for as long as possible and not removed in favor of dental implants. There exists no evidence that any alloplastic tooth replacement including dental implants offers greater service or longevity than a healthy and unrestored or conservatively restored natural tooth.

With hypodontias come the frequent observations of retained deciduous teeth. These deciduous teeth should be strategically retained and in concert with prudent orthodontic therapy (Fig. 4.6). A deciduous tooth with root resorption that is not mobile serves the purpose of maintaining the alveolar bone that is volumetrically important to providing ideal dental implant aesthetics without bone augmentation. The possible ankylosis of a deciduous tooth should be addressed carefully. A high percentage of primary teeth that do not have a permanent successor will ankylose. The value of an ankylosed tooth is again related to maintaining alveolar bone mass. The risk of maintaining an ankylosed tooth is that advancing growth of both the maxillary and mandibular alveolar ridges proceeds beyond the position of the ankylosed tooth, submerging these teeth relative to their adjacent teeth. The management of these teeth must focus on preserving (or creating) the ideal interproximal dimension for the subsequent implant replacement. This might involve minor enameloplasty or disking of deciduous molars proximal surface so that it is approximately the ideal size for the space that will be filled by the implant and prosthetic crown. Primary second molars are on average 1–2 mm larger in their mesial-distal dimension compared with the permanent second premolar that replaces them. Continued restoration to maintain the occlusal (a common problem with ankylosed primary teeth) and/or the mesial and distal contacts with the adjacent teeth can also be necessary to create the optimal future implant space and site. Continued communication and collaboration of the pediatric, orthodontic, and prosthodontic specialist can successfully manage the hypodontia patient with retained deciduous teeth. Additionally, as treatment progresses toward definitive restoration, the likelihood of bone augmentation and implant placement will require the presentation of the patient to the periodontal or oral surgical specialist. The proper interdisciplinary treatment and consideration of retained deciduous teeth is an important part of managing the patient with oligodontia (Fig. 4.6).

Conclusions

Nonsyndromic selective tooth agenesis is sufficiently prevalent that the majority of dentists will recognize this condition among their patients. In many cases, a single missing tooth represents little challenge in its management as the phenotype is not complex and is analogous to any tooth lost to caries or trauma. However, as the severity increases to include multiple teeth, the patient may express greater concern, and more intensive management is required. Here, collaboration involving a prosthodontist with responsibility for definitive restoration as the patient enters adulthood should be sought during the mixed dentition stage. When oligodontias are encountered, the increased number of missing teeth causes greater influence on alveolar bone resorption and broader influences on the ultimate treatment plan. It is of paramount importance to identify possible definitive treatment plans before initiating or completing orthodontic tooth movement. In oligodontias with increasing numbers of missing teeth, an additional goal of therapy is to maintain retained deciduous teeth to aid in alveolar ridge preservation for eventual implants. In these more complex cases, it is especially important to envision the possible definitive treatment plans and to consult with both the prosthodontic and surgical specialists during active orthodontic and adolescent preventive dental therapy. Dental implants are a standard part of treatment in managing such patients. Remarkable aesthetic and functional rehabilitation of the nonsyndromic selective tooth agenesis patient can be achieved when mutual goals of the patient and treatment team are agreed upon and met.

References

1. Ahn Y, Sanderson BW, Klein OD, Krumlauf R. Inhibition of Wnt signaling by Wise (Sostdc1) and negative feedback from Shh controls tooth number and patterning. Development. 2010;137:3221–31.
2. Andersson B, Bergenblock S, Fürst B, Jemt T. Long-term function of single-implant restorations: a 17- to 19-year follow-up study on implant infraposition related to the shape of the face and patients' satisfaction. Clin Implant Dent Relat Res. 2013;15:471–80.
3. Arzoo PS, Klar J, Bergendal, Norderyd J, Dahl N. WNT10A mutations account for 1/4 of population-based isolated oligodontia and show phenotypic correlations. Am J Med Genet. 2014;164A:353–9.
4. Bernard JP, Schatz JP, Christou P, Belser U, Kiliaridis S. Long-term vertical changes of the anterior maxillary teeth adjacent to single implants in young and mature adults. A retrospective study. J Clin Periodontol. 2004;31(11):1024–8.

5. Burzynski NJ, Escobar VH. Classification and genetics of numeric anomalies of dentition. Birth Defects Orig Artic Ser. 1983;19:95–106.

6. Hosseini M, Worsaae N, Schiødt M, Gotfredsen K. A 3-year prospective study of implant-supported, single-tooth restorations of all-ceramic and metal-ceramic materials in patients with tooth agenesis. Clin Oral Implants Res. 2013;24:1078–87.

7. Chen Y, Bei M, Woo I, Satokata I, Maas R. Msx1 controls inductive signaling in mammalian tooth morphogenesis. Development. 1996;122:3035–44.

8. Cluzeau C, Hadj-Rabia S, Jambou M, Mansour S, Guigue P, Masmoudi S, Bal E, Chassaing N, Vincent MC, Viot G, et al. Only four genes (EDA1, EDAR, EDARADD, and WNT10A) account for 90 % of hypohidrotic/anhidrotic ectodermal dysplasia cases. Hum Mutat. 2011;32(1):70–2.

9. Cobourne MT, Sharpe PT. Diseases of the tooth: the genetic and molecular basis of inherited anomalies affecting the dentition. Wiley Interdiscip Rev Dev Biol. 2013;2:183–212. doi:10.1002/wdev.66.

10. Das P, Stockton DW, Bauer C, Shaffer LG, D'Souza R, Wright T, et al. Haploinsufficiency of Pax9 is associated with autosomal dominant hypodontia. Hum Genet. 2002;110:371–6.

11. Han D, Gong Y, Wu H, Zhang X, Yan M, Wang X, et al. Novel EDA mutation resulting in X-linked non-syndromic hypodontia and the pattern of EDA-associated isolated tooth agenesis. Eur J Med Genet. 2008;51:536–46.

12. Heymann HO. The Carolina bridge: a novel interim all-porcelain bonded prosthesis. J Esthet Restor Dent. 2006;18:81–92; discussion 92.

13. Kokich Jr VO, Kinzer GA. Managing congenitally missing lateral incisors. Part I: canine substitution. J Esthet Restor Dent. 2005;17(1):5–10.

14. Mikkola ML. Molecular aspects of hypohidrotic ectodermal dysplasia. Am J Med Genet A. 2009; 149A(9):2031–6.

15. Nieminen P, Arte S, Pirinen S, Peltonen L, Thesleff I. Gene defect in hypodontia: exclusion of MSX1 and MSX2 as candidate genes. Hum Genet. 1995;96:305–8.

16. Polder BJ, Van't Hof MA, Van der Linden FP, Kuijpers-Jagtman AM. A meta-analysis of the prevalence of dental agenesis of permanent teeth. Community Dent Oral Epidemiol. 2004;32:217–26.

17. Peters H, Balling R. Teeth. Where and how to make them. Trends Genet. 1999;15:59–65.

18. Pjetursson BE, Lang NP. Prosthetic treatment planning on the basis of scientific evidence. J Oral Rehabil. 2008;35 Suppl 1:72–9.

19. Qin H, Xu HZ, Xuan K. Clinical and genetic evaluation of a Chinese family with isolated oligodontia. Arch Oral Biol. 2013;5:1180–6.

20. Scheuber S, Hicklin S, Brägger U. Implants versus short-span fixed bridges: survival, complications, patients' benefits. A systematic review on economic aspects. Clin Oral Implants Res. 2012;23 Suppl 6:50–62.

21. Thesleff I, Niemen P. Tooth morphogenesis and cell differentiation. Curr Opin Cell Biol. 1996;8:844–56.

22. Townsend G, Harries EF, Lesot H, Clauss F, Brook A. Morphogenetic fields within the human dentition: a new, clinically relevant synthesis of an old concept. Arch Oral Biol. 2009;54s:s34–44.

23. Vastardis H. The genetics of human tooth agenesis: new discoveries for understanding dental anomalies. Am J Orthod Dentofacial Orthop. 2000;117:650–6.

24. Xuan K, Jin F, Liu YL, Yuan LT, Wen LY, Yang FS, Wang XJ, Wang GH, Jin Y. Identification of a novel missense mutation of MSX1 gene in Chinese family with autosomal-dominant oligodontia. Arch Oral Biol. 2008;53(8):773–9.

25. Chhabra et al: Chhabra N, Goswami M, Chhabra A. Genetic basis of dental agenesis–molecular genetics patterning clinical dentistry. Med Oral Patol Oral Cir Bucal. 2014;19:e112–e119.

26. Galluccio G, Pilotto A.Genetics of dental agenesis: anterior and posterior area of the arch. Eur Arch Paediatr Dent. 2008 ;9:41–45.

27. Kapadia H, Mues G, D'Souza R. Genes affecting tooth morphogenesis. Orthod Craniofac Res. 2007 Nov;10(4):237–44. Review.

28. Jung RE, Zembic A, Pjetursson BE, Zwahlen M, Thoma DS. Systematic review of the survival rate and the incidence of biological, technical, and aesthetic complications of single crowns on implants reported in longitudinal studies with a mean follow-up of 5 years. Clin Oral Implants Res. 2012;23 Suppl 6:2–21.

29. Raes F, Cooper LF, Tarrida LG, Vandromme H, De Bruyn H.A case-control study assessing oral-health-related quality of life after immediately loaded single implants in healed alveolar ridges or extraction sockets. Clin Oral Implants Res. 2012 ;23: 602–608.

Syndromic Hypodontia and Oligodontia: Ectodermal Dysplasias

5

Clark M. Stanford

Abstract

The lack of tooth formation or dental dysmorphic morphology is one of the phenotypes of various forms of the ectodermal dysplasias (ED). Teeth that do form are often altered in shape and contour and occasionally manifest with delayed eruption. The oral health-care team needs to work with affected individuals starting around the first year of life with age-appropriate and staged oral health interventions through adulthood. For most patients with ED, definitive rehabilitation (with or without implant treatment) should be delayed until skeletal maturity. Having said this, starting around age 2–3, pediatric removable prosthesis is appropriate with pediatric dentist-guided care through adulthood. As a part of the final reconstruction as a young adult, the team needs to plan for maintenance issues and complications and use a defined set of diagnostic risk factors in the assessment of the affected individual. Through careful assessment, planning, good team communication, and partnership with the affected individual and her/his family, a successful long-term solution can be developed that provides the best in patient-oriented outcomes.

Introduction

A variety of hereditary conditions are associated with teeth that are missing due to developmental failure (e.g., Down syndrome, ectodermal dysplasias). Clinicians should consider the possible existence of a syndrome if an individual is congenitally missing teeth, and as the number of missing teeth increases, the likelihood that the condition is syndrome associated increases. If an undiagnosed syndrome is suspected, then referral to an appropriate health-care provider (e.g., physician, medical geneticist) for evaluation should be discussed with the patient or parent. The ectodermal dysplasias (EDs) are a diverse set of syndromic conditions derived from mutations affecting a variety of important developmental pathways including communication between the overlaying ectoderm and the underlying mesoderm in

A chapter submission for "Craniofacial and Dental Developmental Defects – Diagnosis and Management" – Dr. Tim Wright, editor

C.M. Stanford, DDS, PhD
The University of Illinois at Chicago,
801 South Paulina Street,
102c (MC621), Chicago, IL 60612, USA
e-mail: cmstan60@uic.edu

embryonic development. Conventionally, a clinical definition of the phenotype has been for individuals in which two or more ectodermally derived structures (e.g., hair, teeth, nails, sweat glands, feathers, etc.) are affected. The structures either do not form (aplasia) or have altered phenotypes (dysplasias) such as conical-shaped or microdontic teeth [1]. Originally described in its current classification by Freire-Maia and Pinheiro, the most common form of ED syndromes is referred to as X-linked hypohidrotic ectodermal dysplasia or HED (but note that there are more than 200 types of ED with widely different phenotypes) [2]. The X-linked HED phenotype is often defined by a combination of features including hypodontia (missing <5 teeth), oligodontia (missing six or more teeth), and, rarely, anodontia (missing all teeth); conical-shaped teeth; altered hair growth, distribution, and amount (trichodysplasia); reduced sweating (dyshidrosis) in some forms; altered mucosal sebaceous function (asteatosis) leading to dry mucosal surfaces and significant mucosal crusting; and altered keratin nail formation in some types (onychodysplasia) (Fig. 5.1).

In regard to the dental malformations, the largest physiological issues are loss of function, lack of alveolar ridge development, arch length tooth size discrepancies, and hyposalivation. The latter can place the patient at a high risk of dental decay. The North American National Foundation for Ectodermal Dysplasias (www.NFED.org) has led an effort to create a consensus on timing, dental therapy, and realistic approaches to oral rehabilitation in children and young adults affected with the EDs. These guidelines outline tooth replacement therapy that is both fixed to teeth and removable with or without oral implant options. Implant therapy is primarily for the skeletally mature adult [3–8]. A leading principle of these guidelines is to provide age-appropriate therapies that holistically respect the integrity of the patient and cultural competency and provide staged therapies allowing the patient to adapt to each approach as they are undergoing what growth potential they have [9–11]. Note also, in this discussion, that it is often better to use the medical term "care plan" rather than "treatment plan" since the latter suggests something is

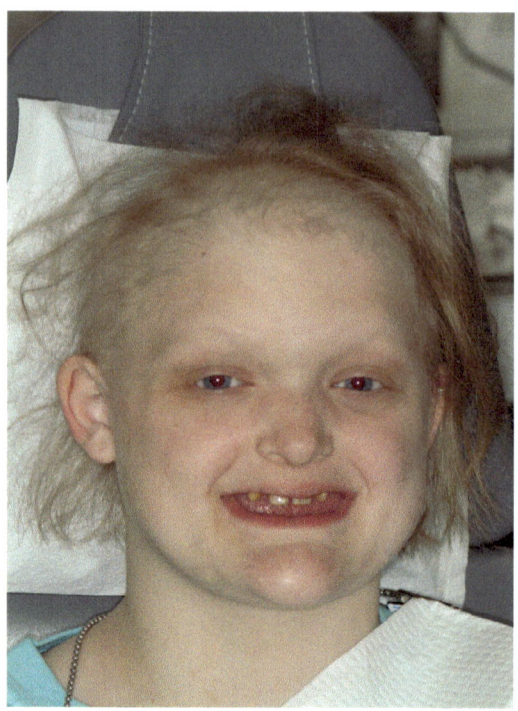

Fig. 5.1 Affected female patient with X-linked hypohidrotic ectodermal dysplasia (HED) demonstrating many of the phenotypic features of HED including alopecia, dry skin, thin nose, prominent chin point, periorbital pigmentation, etc. Carrier females with X-linked HED often demonstrate a range of phenotypic expression depending on when X-inactivation occurs during development

needed (when it may not) and indicates the long-term interests of the patient and their holistic perceived outcomes of care are more important (patient-centric care) than any clinical perception of care or the superiority thereof [10–16].

In the young child (age 0–6), a care plan involving removable prosthesis can usually be considered around the age of 3 (shortly after being potty trained, a relative perception of body awareness). Any young child should see a dentist by the age of 1 (American Academy of Pediatric Dentistry recommendations), and if multiple teeth are missing, a potential diagnosis of one of the ectodermal dysplasias should be contemplated (Fig. 5.2). A pediatric dentist is often the lead consultant although it may be useful to consult with a prosthodontist who is comfortable managing the affected individual as an adult. In this way, the affected individual builds a bond of

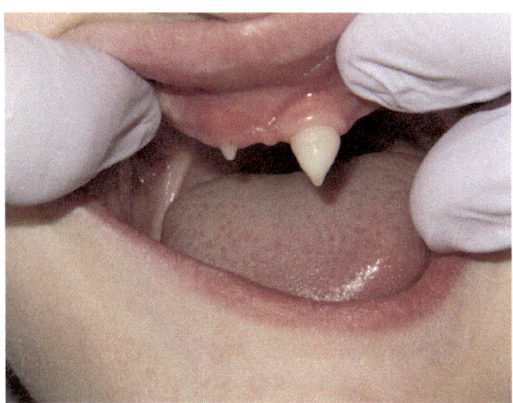

Fig. 5.2 Common presenting oral condition in the X-linked HED including multiple missing teeth (oligodontia); sharp, pointed incisal development of the central incisors; and thin or aplastic ridge development

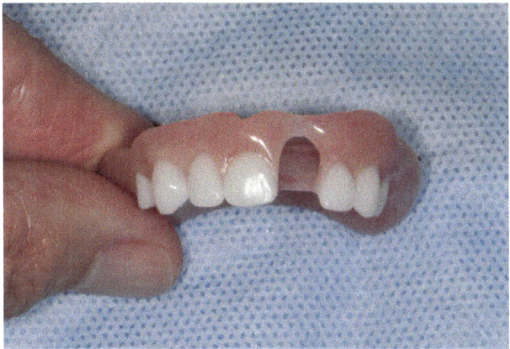

Fig. 5.3 Denture fabrication in the young child is limited to complete or simple acrylic partial dentures with space provided to allow continued eruption of the teeth

trust with the entire care team and there is a better transition of care as they reach adulthood. At the initial appointment, an exam of the number and shape of the current erupted teeth should be made along with palpation of tooth buds. The integrity of the palate and the degree of salivation should be noted. Generally a removable or pediatric fixed prosthesis can be considered (Fig. 5.3) [6]. This is usually performed by a pediatric dentist and/or coordinated with a prosthodontist. The dentures and denture teeth need to be age appropriate in shape, size, and dimensions [17, 18]. If a partial or overdenture approach is used, the parents/caregiver has to be sure to clean the retainer teeth thoroughly on a daily basis and to consider the use of aggressive preventive therapies (e.g., 5 %

NaF varnish). If decalcification occurs on the primary teeth, composite resin, zirconium, stainless steel, or related crowns may be indicated. Note that with HED, the incisors and canines often erupt with very sharp fang-like shapes (Fig. 5.2). In this case, the most conservative approach is to bond composite and dome these either as overdenture abutments or fashion the crown shape into an age-appropriate dimension.

In the young child, the prosthetic steps are often simplified relative to the adult complete or partial denture approaches due to timing, need for replacement, resources, and patient tolerance. In a young patient presenting with multiple missing primary and permanent teeth, making a final impression, often with a well-fitting stock tray and a fast setting impression material (e.g., occlusal registration material), may be sufficient. It is also useful to have a pediatric dentist as the lead of the care team and a prosthodontist in a supporting role. A jaw relationship appointment and delivery appointment typically work with a measurement of the length of the lip in the premaxilla region (vestibule to vermillion border). Pediatric denture teeth (e.g., *milk teeth*, Nissin Dental Products, Japan, distributed in North America through Kilgore International, www.kilgoreinternational.com) are positioned on the trial base and an anterior setup evaluated chairside. Often, in a young child, the upper prosthesis can be made first, allowing a period of accommodation, followed by the lower prosthesis 6–12 months later. It is important to relieve the denture in areas where teeth are erupting, often creating holes in the denture to allow maximum tooth eruption. Recall that it is the eruption of the teeth that creates alveolar bone and is responsible for the development of approximately two thirds of the vertical height of the mid and lower face [19]. The parents/caregiver needs to plan on reline and/or remakes about every 2–3 years while the child is growing.

When the child has reached school age (7–12 years), it is important to transition the dentition from the primary to permanent state, allowing for eruption of what permanent teeth will form. Typically, patients will develop certain permanent teeth more often than others (e.g., central

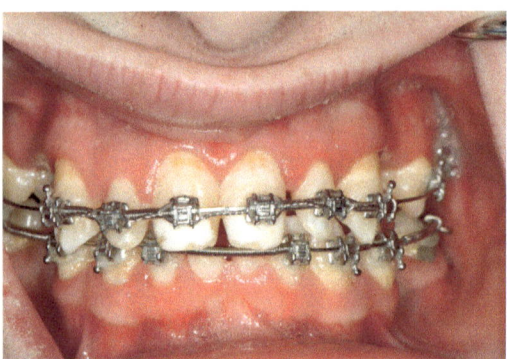

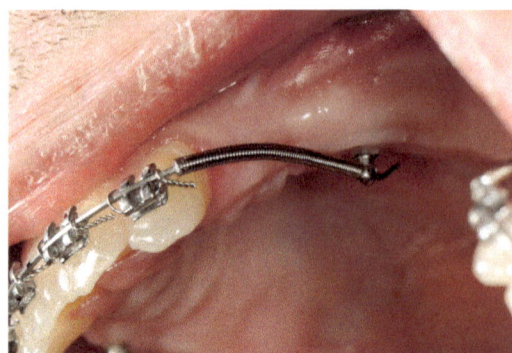

Fig. 5.4 Patient with Witkop's syndrome (tooth and nail syndrome) during orthodontic treatment showing reposition of teeth into a proper position for long-term rehabilitation

Fig. 5.5 In patients missing multiple teeth, temporary anchoring devices (TADs) which are really temporary non-integrating implants are often used during orthodontic therapy

incisors, canines, and first molars). It is important to provide replacement teeth in this population to allow for phonetics, mastication, and social/peer awareness [17, 20, 21]. Typically a more removable approach is used in this population to allow for ongoing growth. This is also a time for orthodontic evaluation, especially as permanent teeth erupt and may need to be guided to proper position (Fig. 5.4). Retained primary teeth should be retained to preserve what alveolar bone has formed. Evaluation for ankylosed primary teeth needs to occur (especially in bounded spaces with permanent teeth on either side). In patients congenitally missing all of their mandibular teeth, consideration may be made for one or two oral implants in the anterior mandible [3]. This should be elected with caution with careful discussion as to why the patient (and not the caregiver) cannot adapt to the lower complete denture. The use of mini-implants (<2 mm diameter) is not commonly considered in this population.

In adolescents to young adults (13 years to maturity), this is an age range when orthodontic therapy should be considered. Comprehensive care in this population should be a team approach between pediatric dentistry, prosthodontics, and orthodontic colleagues. Orthodontic care may be conventional full-banded appliances or assisted with temporary anchoring devices (TADs or "temporary implants") used to support the orthodontic care (Fig. 5.5). These are removed during or at the completion of the orthodontic phase of care. In cases of hypodontia (e.g., missing maxillary lat-

eral incisors), esthetic tooth replacement can be performed either with a removable partial denture, an orthodontic retainer, or a unilateral bonded pontic (Fig. 5.6a–d). In the latter approach, the bonded pontic is typically made with a zirconia core that is either tribochemical silica-based silinated (e.g., Rocatec Bonding System, 3M ESPE, St. Paul, MN) or the TZP ZrO substructure is pressed with a hydrofluoric acid-etchable glass ceramic (e.g., e.max Press, Ivoclar Vivadent, Amherst, NY) and bonded to the mesial aspect of the canine with a veneer-based cement system (e.g., RelyX Veneer, 3M ESPE) [22]. An important goal for the transitional period is a stable, esthetic, and functional dentition without overtreatment or loss of retained primary teeth that are developing or maintaining alveolar bone. It is most important that the maximal potential of craniofacial growth be accomplished during this period.

If denture retention is insufficient, from the patient's perceptive, oral implant therapy can be considered in the edentulous anterior mandible during this period. Although, it is best to plan for a definitive final prosthetic design in selecting the implant sites [18]. It is also preferable to avoid extensive bone grafting for site development in this age period.

Oral rehabilitation in the skeletally mature adult needs to be based on a comprehensive evaluation of systemic health and oral health risk factors with a strong weighting on patient-oriented outcomes, desires, and values. In this population, a multidisciplinary team is critical with additional orthodontic

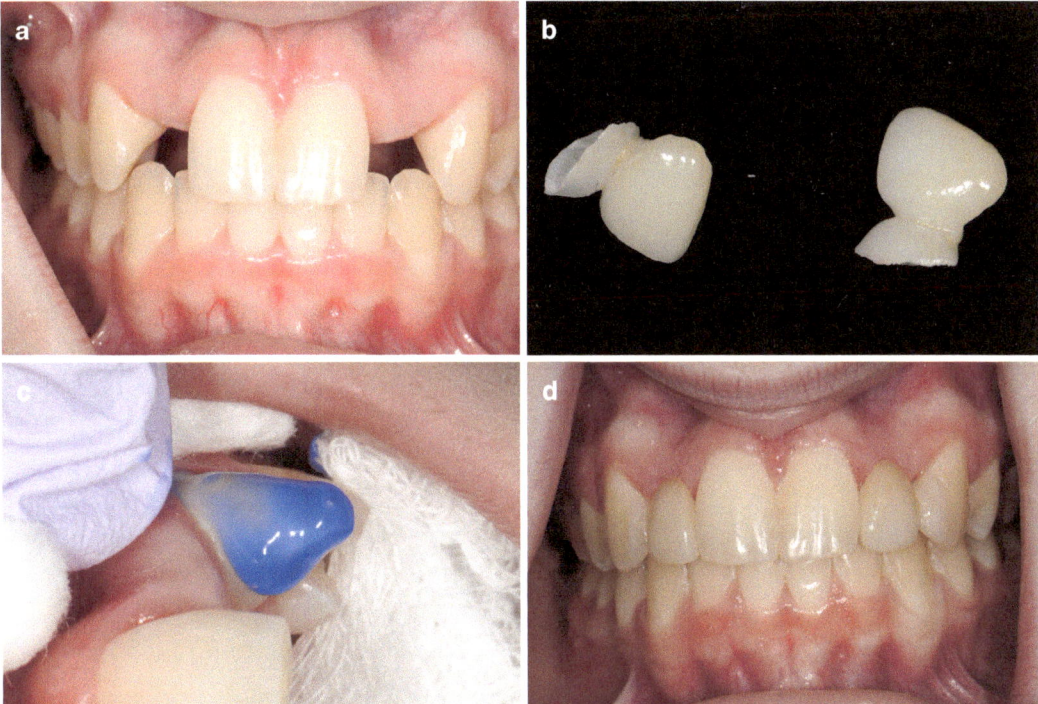

Fig. 5.6 (**a**) A 14-year-old female during post-orthodontic retention phase of care with hypodontia (missing lateral incisors). (**b**) Missing lateral incisors are replaced with zirconia substructure and pressed lithium disilicate pontics adhesively bonded to the mesial aspect of the canines. Note the wrapping support created in the retainer design. (**c**) The retainer teeth are etched and prepared using a conventional veneer bonding system. (**d**) The patient at a 3-year recall with the lateral incisors restored with cantilever pontics bonded to the mesial aspect of the canines allowing ongoing growth of the premaxilla, natural individual tooth eruption, and anterior occlusal stability

and oral surgical phases of care (e.g., Le Fort midface orthognathic procedures). The prosthetic outcomes need to be carefully planned by the prosthodontist and strategic decisions made as to retention of primary (or sometimes permanent) teeth, use of root canal therapy (RCT) and RPD overdentures for multiple missing contiguous teeth, and/or need for extensive bone grafting for a multiple oral implant rehabilitation (Fig. 5.7a–d). In any event, the patient needs to understand that any prosthodontic intervention will have significant maintenance issues and will probably need to be replaced multiple times in the patient's lifetime [12]. The conical or malformed shape of the permanent teeth can be corrected with direct composite bonding or conservative bonded ceramic veneers (partial coverage onlays) based on light surface preparation of the teeth and careful orthodontic planning/spacing to allow optional positioning of the permanent conical-shaped crown in the middle of the planned ceramic veneers (e.g., e.max Press, Ivoclar Vivadent, Amherst, NY) (Fig. 5.8a–f). Oral implant therapy can be very helpful in this population given a proper diagnostic work-up and careful planning is performed. A systematic assessment of risk factors is essential (Table 5.1). Note in Table 5.1 the importance of mucosal tissue thickness and width and the need to use connective tissue grafting (alloplastic or autoplastic) to augment the mucosal tissues in the planned implant sites. In a retrospective survey of 98 patients affected with ED, treated with oral implants at the National Institutes of Health (NIH) in the 1980s, it was observed that a relatively high rate of implant maintenance complications occurred over time [17]. With 56 male and 46 female subjects having 73 % of the implants in the lower jaw, it was noted that 52 % of the implants had complications such as infections, lost implants, loose dentures,

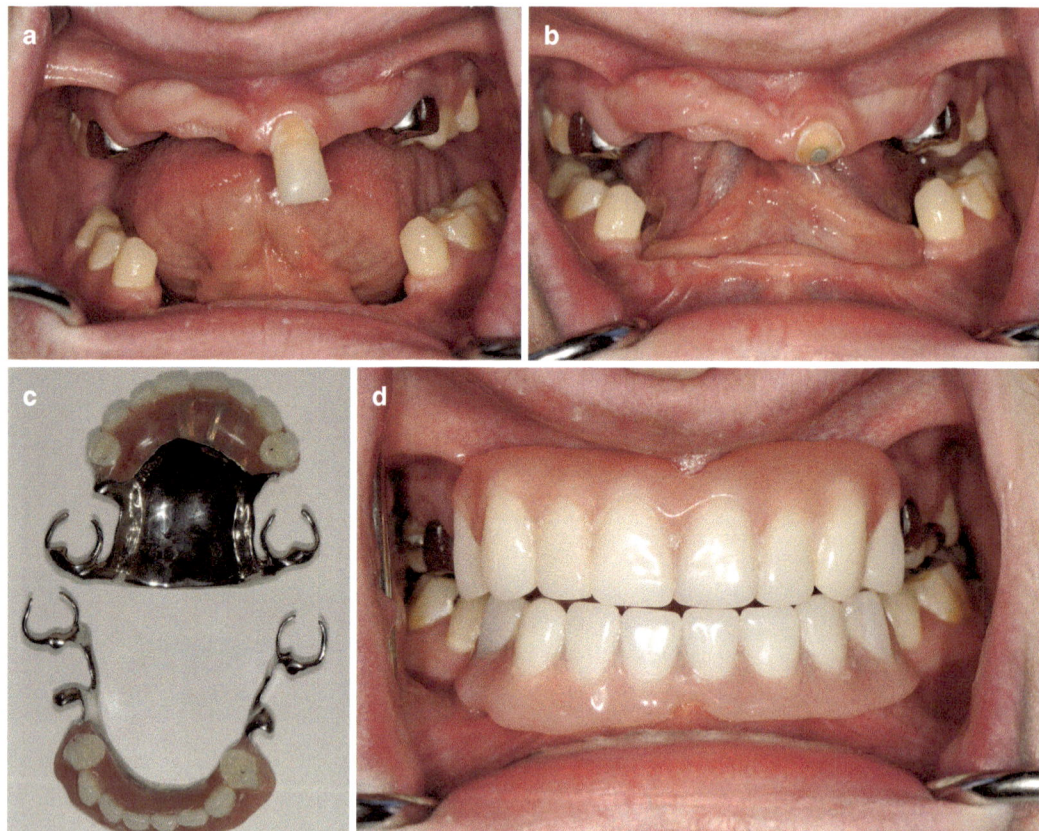

Fig. 5.7 (**a**) A 20-year-old male with HED presents with multiple missing teeth, supraerupted central incisor, ridge aplasia, and retained primary molars restored with stainless steel crowns. Care plan included root canal therapy on the central and conversation to an overdenture abutment under an RPD. (**b**) Patient following RCT and central incisor converted to an overdenture abutment. (**c**) Conventional upper and lower cast partial dentures. The use of RPD is a less expensive approach and rapidly restores the multiple missing teeth for this patient. (**d**) The patient was restored with the upper RPD overdenture and lower RPD. Excellent oral hygiene is very important with this approach due to the high caries risk in the HED population along with the plaque retention that occurs with these types of prosthesis

remakes/relines, and combinations of these complications. It is interesting to note that most of the subjects were happy with the outcomes regardless of the complications. In a study by Bergendal et al. [23], the authors reported on a retrospective study of Nordic regional treatment centers on ED-affected children treated with oral implants between 1985 and 2005 [23]. Twenty-one children, treated with 33 implants due to agenesis or trauma, with a subgroup of ED-affected children (5 treated with 14 implants) at 5–12 years of age were reported. The authors reported that 9 of the 14 implants were lost prior to loading in the ED cohort, warranting caution with the approach and implant system being used at that time [23]. In the Netherlands, a retrospective study following 129 subjects in the Dutch health-care system having tooth agenesis (mostly hypodontia) noted over an observation period of 3–79 months (mean of 46 months in function) that 36 % of subjects had severe orthodontic root resorption, 12 % had significant bone loss (>5 mm), and 57 % had mucosal discoloration around the implant abutments [24]. In our Craniofacial Clinical Research Center at the University of Iowa, we have longitudinally followed 46 subjects with HED or Witkop's syndrome (tooth and nail ectodermal dysplasias). In this population with at least 3–28 years of follow-up, we have 32 subjects treated with corticocancellous hip grafts restored with 231 oral implants (3 different systems, 4 turned surface, 227 moderately rough acid-etched or TiO-blasted surfaces) with fixed or removable options. 80 % were treated with

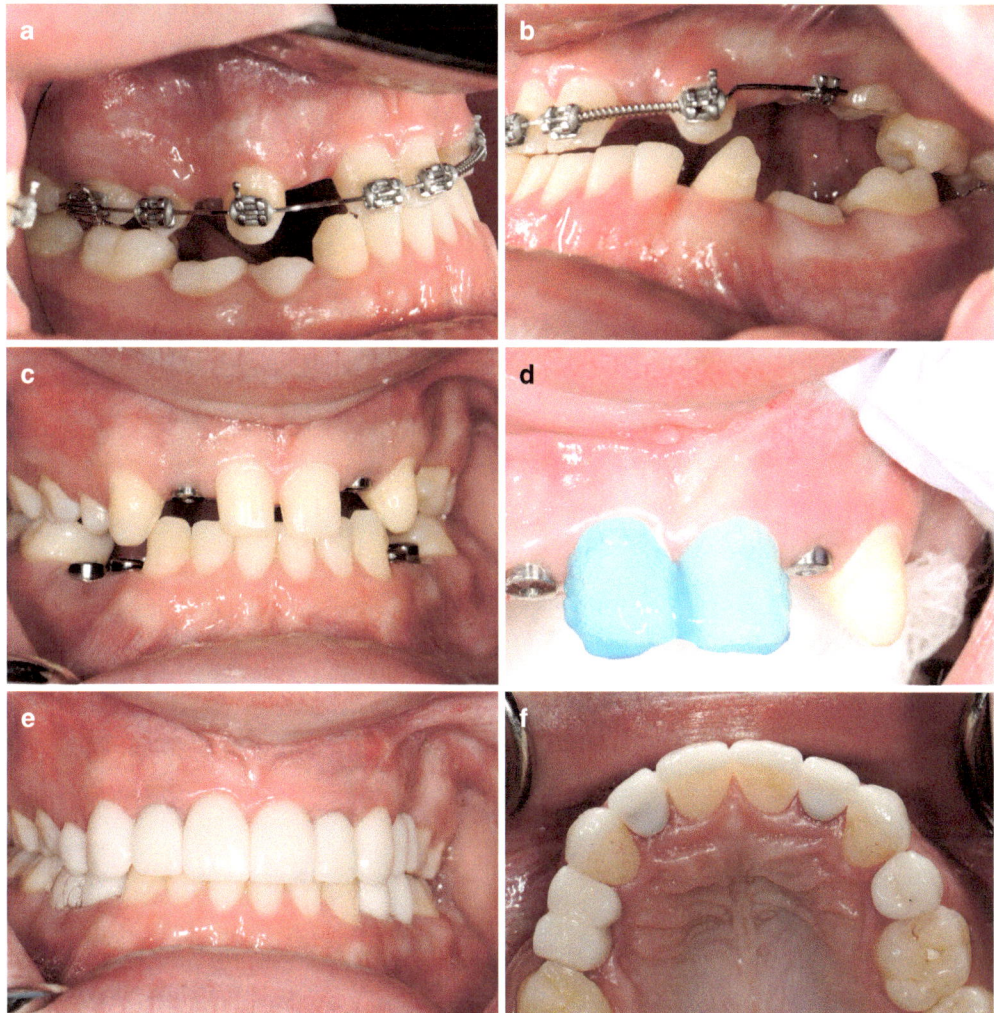

Fig. 5.8 (**a**) A 20-year-old male with Witkop's syndrome presents with retained primary teeth, ankylosed primary teeth, and class III malocclusion with a dental compensation necessitating an orthodontic and orthognathic midface Le Fort I procedure to correct midface asymmetry. (**b**) Patient's occlusion and oligodontia demonstrating both the supraeruption of the lower canine, the distal inclination of the lower incisors, and ankylosed primary teeth (being used for orthodontic anchorage in the maxilla). (**c**) Anterior view of patient's occlusion. Orthodontic positioning of the teeth has set up for ceramic veneers on the remaining permanent teeth. Patient had a Le Fort I midface advancement followed by implant placement. (**d**) Teeth were prepared for the veneers using a conventional three-step adhesive bonding systems. (**e**) Anterior view following restoration (BL3 shade, e.max lithium disilicate, Ivoclar Vivadent, Amherst, NY). (**f**) Occlusal view demonstrating veneers on the canines and central incisors (1 mm flat reduction, light facial and cervical preparation). Maxillary right microdontic first premolar was restored with a ceramic onlay to restore normal contours. Maxillary left premolars restored with one implant and a molar-sized crown shaped as two premolars when viewed from the buccal corridor. Maxillary lateral incisors were restored with implants (3.5 mm ASTRA TECH-TX Implant System, DENTSPLY Implants, Waltham, MA) using CAD/CAM abutment and individual crowns (Gold Hue, Atlantis DENTSPLY Implants, Waltham, MA)

a conventional two-stage healing approach. In this cohort, we have one lost implant at 6 weeks following placement (implant with moderately rough surface, anterior mandible in dense type I bone). We have noticed that 78 % of the hip grafted sites over time develop the same mucosal discoloration reported by the Dutch group, emphasizing that autogenous grafting is useful but not stable and long term and that mucosal thickness augmentation procedures (e.g., connective tissue grafting,

Table 5.1 Guidelines for the evaluation of implant-related risk factors and elements of informed consent

	Guideline	Issue	Management
1	Three-dimensional mucosal biotype?	Thin biotypes (<2 mm thick) are associated with recession and implant bone loss and compromised esthetics. Evaluate for thin bone all around the planned implant site	Consider connective tissue grafting, and consider the thickness of the facial plate of the bone. Plan for at least 1–1.5 mm of bone all around the planned implant. If not, plan for site preservation or development grafting procedures. Use CBCT approaches to evaluate implant sites
2	Symmetry of the smile?	Asymmetry between the anterior and posterior occlusal planes relative to the lips and smile upon activation of the muscles of mastication	Evaluate the posterior occlusal plane relative to the commissures of the lips; evaluate the degree of and asymmetry of the buccal corridor side to side
3	Anterior incisal plane?	Asymmetry in the canine to canine tooth size, arch length discrepancy?	Orthodontic balancing of the anterior incisal edges (prefer lateral incisors to be offset from the central incisor)
		Danger or ongoing passive eruption leading to changes in the incisal edges of the anterior incisal plane	Orthodontic positioning with tight lingual coupling of the maxillary cingulum with the incisal edge of the opposing mandibular incisors. If this cannot be obtained, consider composite resin cingulum stops to prevent nonuniform passive eruption
		Mandibular incisor supraeruption? Anterior natural tooth vertical and horizontal overlap (overjet and overbite)	May need to consider intrusion or extraction of the opposing teeth if function is compromised in the care plan development
4	Tooth to tooth proportions?	Balance of tooth proportions in the anterior incisal plane	Based on central incisor proportions (e.g., 70–75 % of the width relative to the inciso-gingival dimension), if lateral is 2/3 mesial-distal dimension or less, consider cantilever lateral incisor pontics
5	Tooth to tooth relationships?	Asymmetry in canine, lateral and central incisor positions creating nonuniform diastemas	Orthodontic management to allow either reshaping, bonding, or ceramic veneers
6	Gingival position of interproximal contact points?	Asymmetry can lead to interproximal recession or gingival CEJ symmetry issues	Evaluate in provisional restorations, determine if apical position of interproximal contact points needs to be moved more apical
7	Type of defect?	Evaluate the degree of hard and mucosal augmentation that will be needed and the impact on timing of the procedures	Consult patient about timing of procedures relative to major life events, plan for interim restorations needed during healing and for tissue sculpting

Table 5.1 (continued)

	Guideline	Issue	Management
8	History of recession?	Evaluate other sites in the oral cavity for signs of recession	Carefully evaluate especially in post-orthodontic situation, consider augmentation procedures
9	History of defect?	Degree of bone and mucosal defect	In sites with congenitally missing teeth, consider orthodontic augmentation approaches and/or staged surgical procedures
10	Mucosal health?	Mucosal inflammation, especially with interim restorations, complicates final esthetics	Mucosal tissues need to be in optimal health; consider orthodontic extrusion if necessary (esp. in cases of external root resorption)

Adapted from Stanford [18]

use of mucosal thickening agents such as AlloDerm (BioHorizons, Birmingham, AL) or PerioDerm (Symbios, DENTSPLY Implants, Waltham, MA) and dermal matrices) should be considered (Fig. 5.9).

Prosthetic treatment options are diverse for this population as they reach skeletal maturity. While there is some debate as to when oral implant intervention can take place in hypodontia, it is typically considered after the age of 18–20. As described in Table 5.1, key assessments are needed especially in post-orthodontic retention, tooth mobility, and the stability of the occlusion. As a care plan is developed, it is important to engage the affected individual as to personal expectations from these procedures. As a part of the informed consent process, it is important to outline the strengths and challenges of each procedure being proposed (in a language that the patient and caregivers can understand). Health literacy is an important aspect of this process, and it is important to have the caregiver and patient reflect on what is being proposed and articulate back to the care team the elements of the conversation regarding strengths and challenges that they comprehend [25, 26]. Supportive written materials and illustrations are also helpful but are not a substitute for careful, health literacy-appropriate conversations. Alternatives to the proposed care plan should be discussed (including strengths and challenges) as well as reasonable expectations of outcomes if no intervention is done [27].

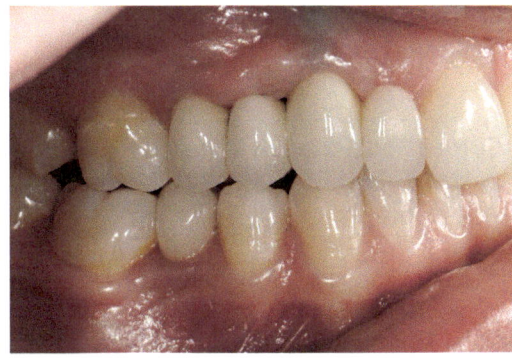

Fig. 5.9 Female patient with Witkop's syndrome at 7-year recall exam. Implants were placed in the maxillary canine region (#6 and #11) with a ramal autogenous graft in the second premolar region (#4 and #13), restored with two FPDs using cantilever pontics for the lateral incisors following the rules presented in Table 5.1. Note the graying of the facial mucosa that was present, a common observation at long-term follow-up indicating resorption of the graft regardless if an implant is placed or not

As the care plan is developed, esthetic and functional outcomes of implant treatment require comprehensive diagnostic and care planning. For many of the affected ED patients, an experienced craniofacial team is often recommended including a pediatric dentist, orthodontist, oral maxillofacial surgeon, periodontist, prosthodontist, laboratory technician, as well as team members such as radiologists and dental and surgical nurses [18]. In some cases it will also be helpful to have a social worker and support from speech pathology. The initial assessment of the patient's medical and dental history is to determine the implant system and devices that will meet the patient's therapeutic and esthetic requirements. The assessment should determine a patient's risks for a surgical intervention especially with some of the P63 variants of ED (e.g., Hay-Wells syndrome, ectodermal dysplasia, ectrodactyly, cleft lip/palate syndrome) in which predictable grafting may be a significant challenge [28]. Throughout the surgical and prosthetic phases of the reconstruction, the dental practitioner should obtain a comprehensive written and verbal informed consent for patient treatment. The care team may find it useful to have a genetic or clinical phenotype diagnosis made by a clinical geneticist (often appointed in the Department of Pediatrics in major medical centers). This can aid in providing supporting data for care plan preauthorizations to insurance carriers.

Suggested Steps to Consider in the Rehabilitation of the Affected Adult Patient

To create a predictable care plan, the prosthodontist should design and compose the proposed prosthesis during the diagnostic phase. For implant-based rehabilitations, planning will dictate the number of implants, size, diameter, and their position and angulation [29, 30]. Based on this diagnostic information, a surgical guide or denture can indicate the desired implant position, angulation, and need for hard/soft tissue augmentation before or during implant placement. During the clinical exam, the dentist should carefully evaluate the residual ridge for its shape and contour. A careful evaluation of the patient's risk factors for soft and hard tissue changes (Table 5.1), whatever final restoration is planned, should be made to encourage realistic patient expectations (Fig. 5.10).

Preoperative planning helps to achieve esthetic goals by ensuring the implant placement is restoratively driven. Implant-retained fixed partial dentures (FPDs) are an excellent alternative to long edentulous spans that conventionally would be restored with removable partial dentures (RPDs). On the other hand, an RPD can be less expensive with fewer risks than a complex surgical intervention. During the informed consent process, care plan alternatives should include a discussion regarding the ability to control esthetics and function with the various methods of tooth replacement including conventional FPDs, adhesive resin restorations ("Maryland" bridges), implants, and/or removable partial dentures.

Fig. 5.10 (**a**) Patient with Witkop's syndrome (tooth and nail syndrome) following completion of the orthodontic phase of care. Note posterior molars in infraocclusion due to upper airway distress syndrome. Patient presented with multiple missing teeth, malformed tooth anatomy, and hypomineralized enamel (variant form of amelogenesis imperfecta). (**b**) Image of patient's fingernails showing the deformed shape and contour common with Witkop's syndrome. (**c, d**) Following mounting at the proposed therapeutic vertical dimension (determined using common prosthetic rule in complete denture therapy such as phonetics and esthetic tooth position), the diagnostic casts then had a full-contoured diagnostic wax-up to plan for the final contours and planned veneers. (**e**) Panoramic image reconstruction from CBCT showing radicular distal angulation of the maxillary canines blocking the restorative space in the premolar region for two adjacent implants. Careful planning and stability of the canines allowed a care plan that involved FPD from one implant placed in the second premolar region and rigidly connected to the canine, bilaterally. (**f**) Occlusal view of zirconia CAD/CAM abutment in the second premolar implant (ATLANTIS, DENTSPLY Implants, Waltham, MA) and the prepared maxillary canine. (**g**) Zirconia-based fixed partial denture trial fitted (Studio 32, Cedar Rapids, Iowa). (**h**) Due to the infra-occluded molars, related to the tongue thrust habit of the upper airway distress syndrome, a ceramic veneer was planned for both mandibular first molars. (**i**) Final lower restorations ready for delivery. Lower jaw had one implant placed in the premolar region with a molar-sized restoration designed to look like two premolars. One implant was placed at the central incisor position with a cantilever pontic. A ceramic onlay was made for each first mandibular molar to bring these into occlusion. (**j**) Lower molar region showing zirconia abutment in place. (**k**) Facial view of completed restorations at 4-year recall. Note mucosal health and lack of reactive infraocclusion. Patient uses a rigid vacuform retainer on a nightly basis. (**l**) Maxillary right incisor region showing mucosal stability around the veneers and retainer on the FPD. (**m**) Maxillary left incisor region showing similar response to the right side. (**n**) Mandibular central incisor region showing 4-year tissue stability with a narrow-diameter implant in the left central incisor region (#25) and a cantilever pontic in the right central incisor region (#26)

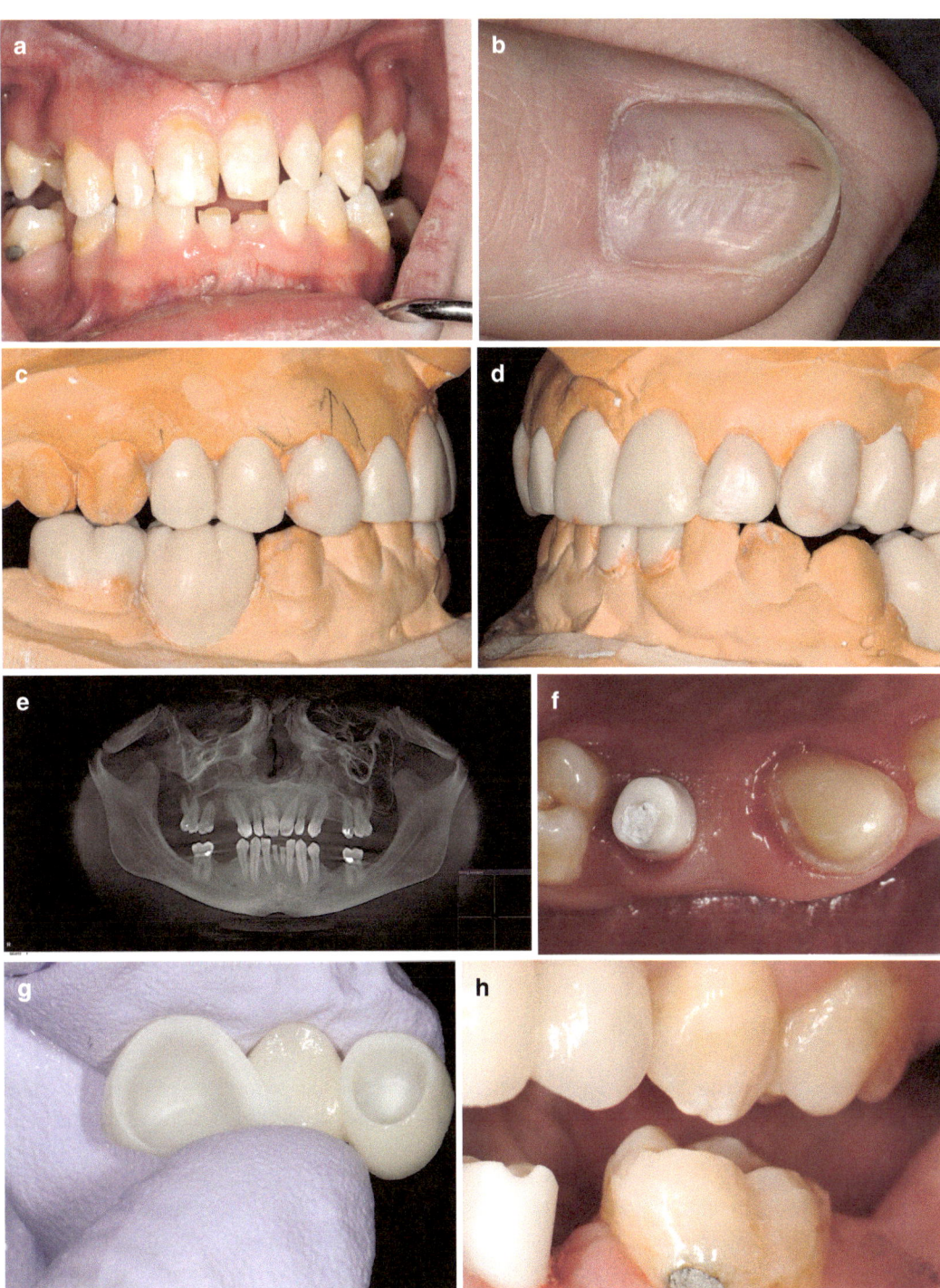

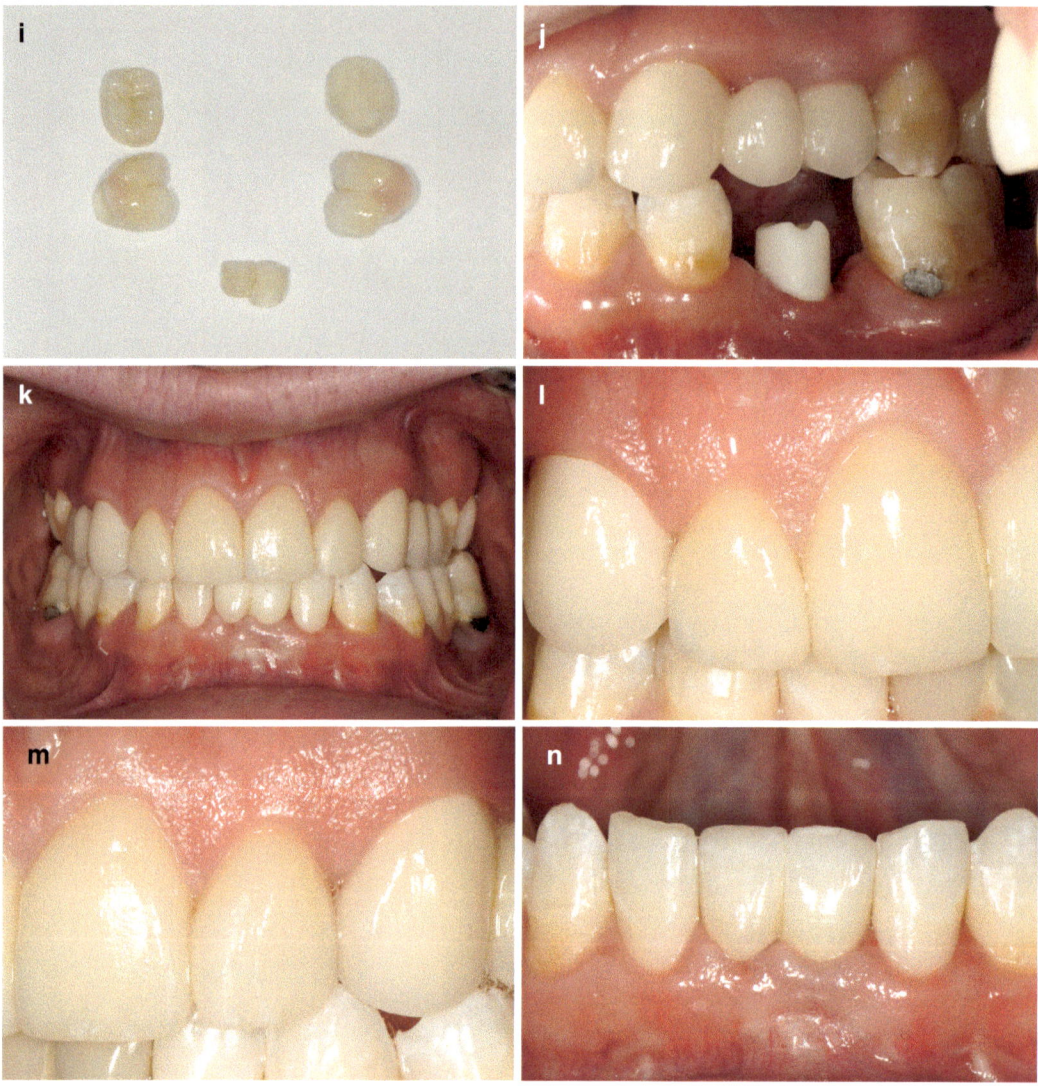

Fig. 5.10 (continued)

The diagnostic phase should determine the number of endosseous-style implants to be placed. When replacing multiple adjacent teeth with dental implants, it is often clinically useful to replace three teeth with a short-span FPD on two implants utilizing the pontic to adjust for contours and final implant position (Fig. 5.10). This approach is especially useful in the anterior maxilla involving multiple teeth where the smallest tooth to be replaced is planned as a pontic (Table 5.1) with implants placed in the canine and central incisor region.

When a tooth or teeth are missing in the anterior region, the dentition tends to be positioned more facially relative to the central axis of the alveolar ridge, resulting in a thin facial plate of bone over the teeth. Upon tooth loss, this facial plate is often unevenly resorbed in a palatal and apical direction (e.g., average of 3–4 mm of bone resorption) in the maxillae [31–36]. The position and stability of the facial/buccal plate of the bone should be considered for any evidence of bone loss, which often occurs in cases involving traumatic fracture or, potentially, during orthodontic therapy. In the mandible, the resorption pattern can occur at an uneven rate causing increased bone loss on the thin superior regions, producing a wider ridge with high muscle attachments. When determining the optimal tooth position for functional and esthetic purposes, create a diagnostic setup with denture teeth on a trial base with soft and hard tissue contours waxed out to full contour. A vacuum-formed matrix of this diagnostic setup can then assist the surgeon in determining the position, placement, and volume of site development (hard and soft tissue grafting) needed for site development [18]. In planning the occlusion, one should consider tooth contacts in centric relation or maximum intercuspation providing vertical loading down the long axis of the implant(s) or controlled loading if tilted implants are to be deployed [37, 38]. Large lateral sliding contacts may create elevated bending or torsional loads leading to premature failure of abutments, fracture of the crown or bridge's mechanical components, and mesial migration of anterior teeth away from posterior implants, opening posterior contact points [39, 40].

Occasionally, implants are placed and connected to natural teeth using an FPD with a rigid or nonrigid connector [22]. Unpredictable incidences of movement (intrusion) of the natural retainer teeth have been reported in cases with use of a nonrigid connector [41, 42]. To provide a prosthesis that is only supported or retained by implants requires placing additional implants and/or augmentation procedures (e.g., onlay bone, sinus lift grafting, distraction osteogenesis, etc.). There are times when a tooth-/implant-supported FPD is the care plan of choice due to lack of anatomic space yet using teeth as retainers that have minimal mobility (Fig. 5.10 series) [43].

Careful oral implant placement in the partially edentulous or single-tooth situation is critical for achieving a predictable esthetic outcome. As described in Table 5.1, the initial evaluation considers factors associated with sufficient bone and soft tissue volume. Additionally, the prosthodontist should discuss these risk factors with the patient and members of the implant team. When evaluating any proposed site in all three dimensions for hard and soft tissue contours, the dentist should rely on clinical observations, mounted diagnostic casts, and a diagnostic wax-up. When evaluating osseous contours, use palpation and sounding with anesthesia (e.g., an endodontic explorer and stopper probed to the periosteum measuring the gingival thickness every few millimeters) coupled with a CBCT radiographic exam having a radiographic guide (a.k.a. scanning prosthesis) with reference markers (e.g., temporary cement painted on the exterior surface, gutta-percha markers, etc.). The evaluation of the soft tissue contours for shape, quantity, texture, and color (Table 5.1) should include noting the parameters observed in the diagnostic wax-up for generation of the radiographic and surgical guides. The periodontal tissues should be in optimal health before implant placement. A thick periodontal tissue biotype typically has thick flattened osseous plates and offers a higher resistance to recession than a thin tissue biotype, especially on the midfacial aspect. In contrast, a thin periodontal tissue biotype, common in the affected ED population, has a thin erythematous periodontium covering a thin or nonexistent alveolar crest that has an increased risk for soft tissue recession [44]. Removal of a tooth in this condition will probably lose the facial plate over time through resorption regardless if an implant is placed. It may be useful to evaluate the gingiva on the contralateral tooth/teeth to consider the size, shape, and color of the interdental papillae, the arcuate form of the free marginal gingiva, and the relative root shape and size (i.e., transition contour of the abutment and restorative emergence profile), along with the width of the attached gingiva and facial root prominence [43, 44]. Consideration should be made to use soft tissue augmentation procedures in sites of thin tissue biotype as previously discussed. Papillae-saving incisions or CBCT-guided flapless surgical approaches may improve the predictability of implant soft tissue management. However, because the gingival response can be difficult to predict preoperatively, it is important to conduct careful evaluation with informed consent. In situations that pose a high risk of gingival reces-

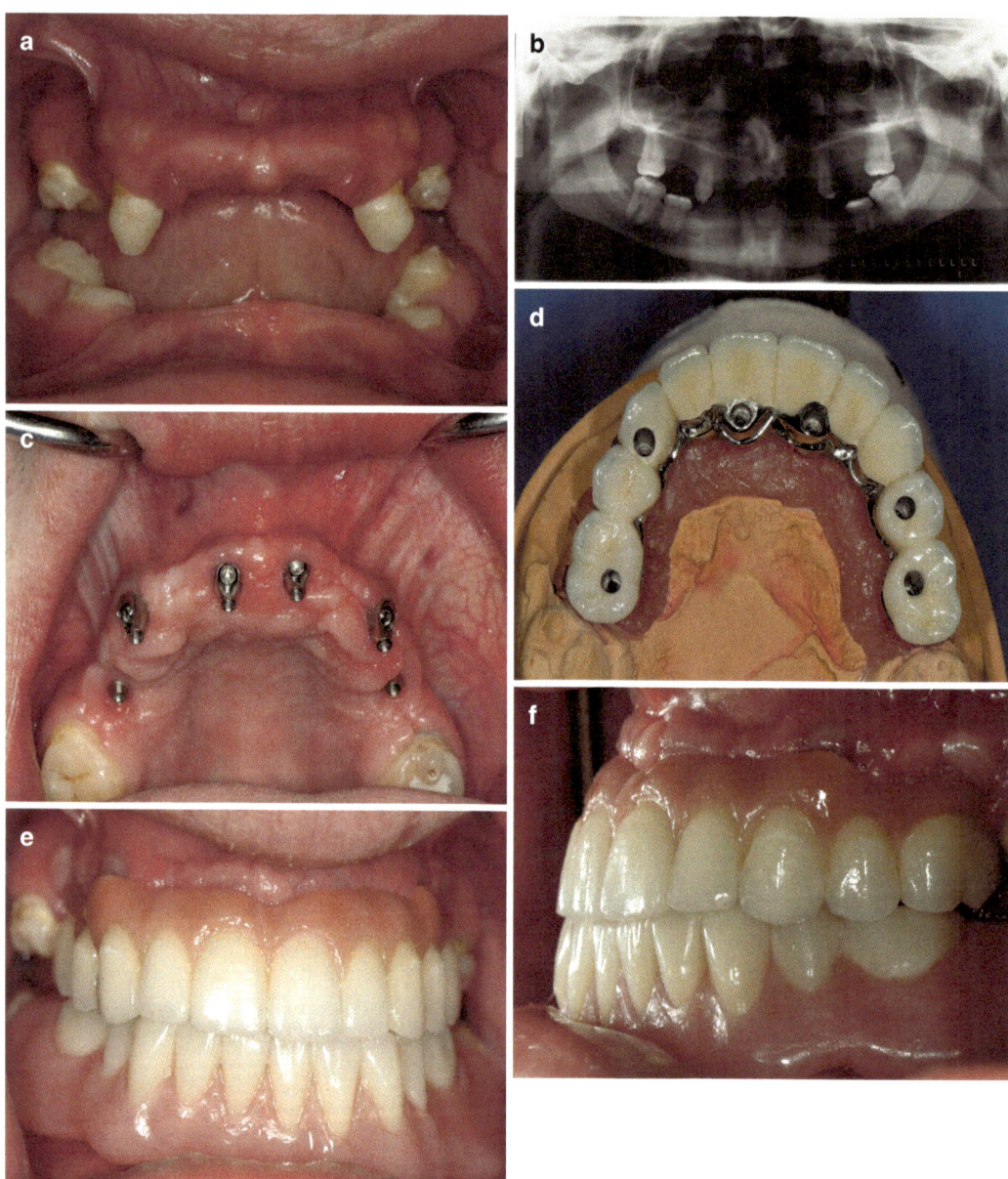

Fig. 5.11 (**a**) Patient presents with X-linked HED as a 21-year-old missing all maxillary permanent premolars, canines, and incisors. Patient is also missing his lower premolars, canines, and incisors. (**b**) Radiographic evaluation notes sufficient osseous anatomy for a fixed upper and lower implant-supported overdenture therapy. (**c**) Six implants are placed and angulated abutments used for a screw-retained approach for the fixed upper prosthesis. (**d**) PFM-FPD screw-retained prosthesis on master cast.

(**e**) Completed prosthesis at 10-year recall using a screw-retained upper prosthesis and a lower overdenture (Locator, Zest Anchors, Escondido, CA). (**f**) Lateral view of reconstruction at 10-year recall. Screw-retained approach allows for maintenance and hygiene therapy. In general, a design concept of ceramic reconstruction in the maxilla and acrylic resin teeth in the mandible reduces chipping and fracture common with ceramic to ceramic reconstructions

sion, a screw-retained crown or prosthesis should be considered instead of a cemented prosthesis (Fig. 5.11 series). This approach allows contours to be retrieved and modified at a later date.

Single-tooth implant applications require adequate interproximal bone related to the restorative space. This concept is articulated in what is referred to as the "rule of six" [30]. For example, a 4-mm-diameter implant requires (1) a minimum of 6 mm of interradicular space, (2) 6 mm mesial-distal space, (3) 6 mm buccal-lingual dimension, (4) minimum of 6 mm space from the opposing occlusal plane to the alveolar crest, (5) coronal-apico distance to safely allow at least a 6-mm-long implant (accounting for the typical 0.5–1 mm additional length created by the rake angle on the end of the drills used to prepare the osteotomy), and (6) an implant placed with the head of the implant 3 mm below the planned midfacial CEJ and the facial aspect to the implant body 2 mm to the lingual or palatal aspect of the planned midfacial CEJ's zenith (a.k.a. "$3 \times 2 = 6$"). Why? During initial healing, at least 1 mm of peri-implant bone continuously models or remodels [45, 46]. For proper development of the emergence profile and the contour of the restoration from the margin through the gingival tissues, the implant should be positioned apical to the adjacent teeth (Fig. 5.8). First, consider the position of the soft tissue thickness and interdental alveolar bone morphology adjacent to the teeth on either side of the proposed site [47, 48]. Proper crown-down implant placement allows the connective tissue and junctional epithelial *biological width* to form on the transmucosal portion of the implant body or on the abutment's mucosal transition zone [49]. At the same time, it is important to avoid excessive countersinking of the implant since this can lead to bone loss, diminish soft tissue support, and increase the risk of long-term gingival recession [50]. If the head of the implant cannot be placed 2–3 mm below the planned CEJ (e.g., due to the proximity of a sinus or vital structure), then a phased treatment may be indicated with bone augmentation, followed later by implant placement or use of an alternative prosthetic intervention. If the tooth was maloccluded or periodontally involved, the tooth's position may not be the optimal position for an implant. In considering immediate placement into an extraction socket, it is often advantageous to position the implant to the palatal aspect of the socket so as the cutting threads of the implant do not cut away or otherwise disrupt the thin facial plate of the bone. This will leave up to 1 mm of space between the implant and the internal surface of the facial bony plate which will fill with the clot. Recently a number of authors have suggested that the facial gap should be filled with a non-resorbing xenograft material and a protective membrane. To establish primary stability with an immediate placement, one third to one half of the implant body should be placed into sound bone that extends beyond the apex of the socket. As a result, the head of the implant may be excessively countersunk (with the associated risk of unpredictable gingival recession). An alternative to immediate extraction is tissue expansion by decorticalization of the crown of the tooth followed by advancement of a facial flap with or without a submucosal connective tissue graft and primary closure. At a later time, the site is reentered and an implant placed in the optimal location. Alternatively, the use of fixed orthodontic extrusion in cases with thicker biotypes can create simple orthodontic luxation of the remaining root or development of additional soft and/or hard tissue, depending on the rate of extrusion [51–53]. Surgical management of the implant site and prosthetic abutment choices affect the preservation, development, and maintenance of the interproximal papillae. In the anterior esthetic zone, a narrow-diameter-healing abutment allows for the provisional crown to reposition the soft tissue at the time of abutment placement. A restoration fabricated at the time of implant placement (immediate provisionalization) can guide the healing of adjacent soft tissues, although the provisional crown should be left out of occlusion (maximum intercuspation and all eccentric positions) during the healing phase. When performing an immediate provisionalization protocol, the occlusion should be monitored because the mobility of the adjacent natural teeth increases during the inflammation and healing of the implant site [54]. Final impressions can be made and the definitive restoration placed after a healing period between 6 and 12 weeks. As hard and soft tissues heal, interproximal contacts and gingival embrasure form allows the maturing tissue to adapt to the provisional restoration(s). Completion of the final restoration can proceed when the gingival tissues have matured, typically 6 weeks or more post placement.

Conclusions

Providing tooth replacement therapy for congenitally missing teeth plays a strong role in the physiological, emotional, and physiological support of our patients. Understanding and conveying the strengths and challenges of the proposed care plan are a vital part of the health literacy process. Oral health-care needs to start in the first year of life and interdisciplinary care is needed between all of the oral health specialties as the patient moves from childhood, through adolescence, and into adulthood. An important underlying feature is to provide care without excessively being aggressive and allow the patient to continue to have as many oral health options as possible throughout their life.

References

1. Carmichael RP, Sandor GK. Use of dental implants in the management of syndromal oligodontia. Atlas Oral Maxillofac Surg Clin North Am. 2008;16(1):33–47.
2. Freire-Maia N, Pinheiro M. Ectodermal dysplasias – some recollections and a classification. Birth Defects Orig Artic Ser. 1988;24(2):3–14.
3. Paulus C, Martin P. Hypodontia due to ectodermal dysplasia: rehabilitation with very early dental implants. Rev Stomatol Chir Maxillofac Chir Orale. 2013;114(3):e5–8.
4. Diz P, Scully C, Sanz M. Dental implants in the medically compromised patient. J Dent. 2013;41(3):195–206.
5. Al-Ibrahim HA, Al-Hadlaq SM, Abduljabbar TS, Al-Hamdan KS, Abdin HA. Surgical and implant-supported fixed prosthetic treatment of a patient with ectodermal dysplasia: a case report. Spec Care Dentist. 2012;32(1):1–5.
6. Bidra AS, Martin JW, Feldman E. Complete denture prosthodontics in children with ectodermal dysplasia: review of principles and techniques. Compend Contin Educ Dent. 2010;31(6):426–33; quiz 34, 44.
7. Van Sickels JE, Raybould TP, Hicks EP. Interdisciplinary management of patients with ectodermal dysplasia. J Oral Implantol. 2010;36(3):239–45.
8. Cronin Jr RJ, Oesterle LJ. Implant use in growing patients. Treatment planning concerns. Dent Clin N Am. 1998;42(1):1–34.
9. Yap AK, Klineberg I. Dental implants in patients with ectodermal dysplasia and tooth agenesis: a critical review of the literature. Int J Prosthodont. 2009;22(3):268–76.
10. Klineberg I, Cameron A, Hobkirk J, Bergendal B, Maniere MC, King N, et al. Rehabilitation of children with ectodermal dysplasia. Part 2: an international consensus meeting. Int J Oral Maxillofac Implants. 2013;28(4):1101–9.
11. Klineberg I, Cameron A, Whittle T, Hobkirk J, Bergendal B, Maniere MC, et al. Rehabilitation of children with ectodermal dysplasia. Part 1: an international Delphi study. Int J Oral Maxillofac Implants. 2013;28(4):1090–100.
12. Bassi F, Carr AB, Chang TL, Estafanous EW, Garrett NR, Happonen RP, et al. Economic outcomes in prosthodontics. Int J Prosthodont. 2013;26(5):465–9.
13. Bassi F, Carr AB, Chang TL, Estafanous EW, Garrett NR, Happonen RP, et al. Psychologic outcomes in implant prosthodontics. Int J Prosthodont. 2013;26(5):429–34.
14. Bassi F, Carr AB, Chang TL, Estafanous EW, Garrett NR, Happonen RP, et al. Functional outcomes for clinical evaluation of implant restorations. Int J Prosthodont. 2013;26(5):411–8.
15. Bassi F, Carr AB, Chang TL, Estafanous E, Garrett NR, Happonen RP, et al. Clinical outcomes measures for assessment of longevity in the dental implant literature: ORONet approach. Int J Prosthodont. 2013;26(4):323–30.
16. Bassi F, Carr AB, Chang TL, Estafanous E, Garrett NR, Happonen RP, et al. Oral Rehabilitation Outcomes Network-ORONet. Int J Prosthodont. 2013;26(4):319–22.
17. Stanford CM, Guckes A, Fete M, Srun S, Richter MK. Perceptions of outcomes of implant therapy in patients with ectodermal dysplasia syndromes. Int J Prosthodont. 2008;21(3):195–200.
18. Stanford CM. Application of oral implants to the general dental practice. J Am Dent Assoc. 2005;136(8):1092–100; quiz 165–6.
19. De Coster PJ, Marks LA, Martens LC, Huysseune A. Dental agenesis: genetic and clinical perspectives. J Oral Pathol Med. 2009;38(1):1–17.
20. Kohli R, Levy S, Kummet CM, Dawson DV, Stanford CM. Comparison of perceptions of oral health-related quality of life in adolescents affected with ectodermal dysplasias relative to caregivers. Spec Care Dentist. 2011;31(3):88–94.
21. Stanford CM, Wagner W, Rodriguez YBR, Norton M, McGlumphy E, Schmidt J. Evaluation of the effectiveness of dental implant therapy in a practice-based network (FOCUS). Int J Oral Maxillofac Implants. 2010;25(2):367–73.
22. Ozkurt Z, Kazazoglu E. Clinical success of zirconia in dental applications. J Prosthodont. 2010;19(1):64–8.
23. Bergendal B, Ekman A, Nilsson P. Implant failure in young children with ectodermal dysplasia: a retrospective evaluation of use and outcome of dental implant treatment in children in Sweden. Int J Oral Maxillofac Implants. 2008;23(3):520–4.
24. Dueled E, Gotfredsen K, Trab Damsgaard M, Hede B. Professional and patient-based evaluation of oral

rehabilitation in patients with tooth agenesis. Clin Oral Implants Res. 2009;20(7):729–36.
25. Gong DA, Lee JY, Rozier RG, Pahel BT, Richman JA, Vann Jr WF. Development and testing of the Test of Functional Health Literacy in Dentistry (TOFHLiD). J Public Health Dent. 2007;67(2):105–12.
26. Richman JA, Lee JY, Rozier RG, Gong DA, Pahel BT, Vann Jr WF. Evaluation of a word recognition instrument to test health literacy in dentistry: the REALD-99. J Public Health Dent. 2007;67(2):99–104.
27. Chalmers I. Well informed uncertainties about the effects of treatments. BMJ. 2004;328(7438):475–6.
28. Monti P, Russo D, Bocciardi R, Foggetti G, Menichini P, Divizia MT, et al. EEC- and ADULT-associated TP63 mutations exhibit functional heterogeneity toward P63 responsive sequences. Hum Mutat. 2013;34(6):894–904.
29. Patzelt SB, Bahat O, Reynolds MA, Strub JR. The all-on-four treatment concept: a systematic review. Clin Implant Dent Relat Res. 2013. doi: 10.1111/cid.12068. [Epub ahead of print]
30. Cooper LF, Pin-Harry OC. "Rules of Six" – diagnostic and therapeutic guidelines for single-tooth implant success. Compend Contin Educ Dent. 2013;34(2): 94–8, 100–1; quiz 2, 17.
31. Sanz M, Cecchinato D, Ferrus J, Salvi GE, Ramseier C, Lang NP, et al. Implants placed in fresh extraction sockets in the maxilla: clinical and radiographic outcomes from a 3-year follow-up examination. Clin Oral Implants Res. 2014;25:321–7.
32. Lindhe J, Bressan E, Cecchinato D, Corra E, Toia M, Liljenberg B. Bone tissue in different parts of the edentulous maxilla and mandible. Clin Oral Implants Res. 2013;24(4):372–7.
33. Januario AL, Duarte WR, Barriviera M, Mesti JC, Araujo MG, Lindhe J. Dimension of the facial bone wall in the anterior maxilla: a cone-beam computed tomography study. Clin Oral Implants Res. 2011;22(10):1168–71.
34. Araujo MG, Lindhe J. Socket grafting with the use of autologous bone: an experimental study in the dog. Clin Oral Implants Res. 2011;22(1):9–13.
35. Huynh-Ba G, Pjetursson BE, Sanz M, Cecchinato D, Ferrus J, Lindhe J, et al. Analysis of the socket bone wall dimensions in the upper maxilla in relation to immediate implant placement. Clin Oral Implants Res. 2010;21(1):37–42.
36. Tomasi C, Sanz M, Cecchinato D, Pjetursson B, Ferrus J, Lang NP, et al. Bone dimensional variations at implants placed in fresh extraction sockets: a multi-level multivariate analysis. Clin Oral Implants Res. 2010;21(1):30–6.
37. Stanford CM. Issues and considerations in dental implant occlusion: what do we know, and what do we need to find out? J Calif Dent Assoc. 2005;33(4):329–36.
38. Klineberg I, Murray G. Osseoperception: sensory function and proprioception. Adv Dent Res. 1999;13:120–9.
39. Goodacre CJ, Kan JY, Rungcharassaeng K. Clinical complications of osseointegrated implants. J Prosthet Dent. 1999;81(5):537–52.
40. Papaspyridakos P, Chen CJ, Chuang SK, Weber HP, Gallucci GO. A systematic review of biologic and technical complications with fixed implant rehabilitations for edentulous patients. Int J Oral Maxillofac Implants. 2012;27(1):102–10.
41. English CE. Biomechanical concerns with fixed partial dentures involving implants. Implant Dent. 1993;2(4):221–42.
42. Rieder CE, Parel SM. A survey of natural tooth abutment intrusion with implant-connected fixed partial dentures. Int J Periodontics Restorative Dent. 1993; 13(4):334–47.
43. Stanford CM, Maze G. Prosthetic considerations for implant surgery. Pract Proced Aesthet Dent. 2006; 18(5):suppl 8.
44. Olsson M, Gunne J, Astrand P, Borg K. Bridges supported by free-standing implants versus bridges supported by tooth and implant. A five-year prospective study. Clin Oral Implants Res. 1995;6(2):114–21.
45. Stanford CM, Brand RA. Toward an understanding of implant occlusion and strain adaptive bone modeling and remodeling. J Prosthet Dent. 1999;81(5): 553–61.
46. Garetto LP, Chen J, Parr JA, Roberts WE. Remodeling dynamics of bone supporting rigidly fixed titanium implants: a histomorphometric comparison in four species including humans. Implant Dent. 1995;4(4):235–43.
47. Bidra AS. Three-dimensional esthetic analysis in treatment planning for implant-supported fixed prosthesis in the edentulous maxilla: review of the esthetics literature. J Esthet Restor Dent. 2011;23(4):219–36.
48. Kan JY, Rungcharassaeng K, Liddelow G, Henry P, Goodacre CJ. Periimplant tissue response following immediate provisional restoration of scalloped implants in the esthetic zone: a one-year pilot prospective multicenter study. J Prosthet Dent. 2007;97 (6 Suppl):S109–18.
49. Berglundh T, Lindhe J. Dimension of the periimplant mucosa. Biological width revisited. J Clin Periodontol. 1996;23(10):971–3.
50. Stanford CM. Achieving and maintaining predictable implant esthetics through the maintenance of bone around dental implants. Compend Contin Educ Dent. 2002;23(9 Suppl 2):13–20.
51. LeSage BP, Lindeboom JA, Tjiook Y, Kroon FH, Spangberg LS, Tozum TF, et al. Improving implant aesthetics: prosthetically generated papilla through tissue modeling with composite. Pract Proced Aesthet Dent. 2006;18(4):257–63.
52. Yeo AB, Cheok CB. Management strategies of the unsalvageable tooth. Dent Update. 2006;33(1):7–8,10–2.
53. Adolfi D, de Freitas AJ, Groisman M. Achieving aesthetic success with an immediate-function implant and customized abutment and coping. Pract Proced Aesthet Dent. 2005;17(9):649–54.
54. Gapski R, Wang HL, Mascarenhas P, Lang NP. Critical review of immediate implant loading. Clin Oral Implants Res. 2003;14(5):515–27.

Diagnosis and Management of Defects of Enamel Development

6

W. Kim Seow and J. Timothy Wright

Abstract

The development of dental enamel can be adversely affected by environmental factors and by alterations in the genes important to normal enamel formation or metabolic changes encountered in some inherited conditions. In addition, the etiology of some enamel defects, such as molar-incisor hypomineralization (MIH), is likely to involve both environmental and hereditary factors. Genetic mutations in the proteins involved in enamel formation may result in a group of conditions known as amelogenesis imperfecta (AI). AI may present clinically as hypoplastic defects which may be expressed as thin or missing enamel, as pits and grooves, or as hypocalcified or hypomature enamel which is discolored and relatively soft and weak. Although the traditional diagnosis of AI is based mainly on the clinical appearance of the defects, the genotypes of many AI phenotypes have now been identified. Many hypoplastic autosomal dominant AI mutations are now known to be associated with changes in *ENAM* or *AMELX* genes which encode for proteins essential for the formation and processing of the matrix for normal mineralization and maturation of enamel. In contrast, the hypocalcified and hypomaturation autosomal recessive AI phenotypes have been associated with mutations in the genes coding for enzymes kallikrein-4 (*KLK4*) and metalloproteinase (*MMP20*), as well as the proteins *FAM83H* and *WDR72*. In addition to AI, there are about 80 hereditary syndromes that can have enamel defects with hypoplastic enamel being the most common phenotype.

W.K. Seow (✉)
Centre for Pediatric Dentistry,
School of Dentistry, The University of Queensland,
Brisbane, QLD, Australia
e-mail: k.seow@uq.edu.au

J.T. Wright
Department of Pediatric Dentistry,
University of North Carolina School of Dentistry,
Chapel Hill, NC, USA

J.T. Wright (ed.), *Craniofacial and Dental Developmental Defects: Diagnosis and Management*,
DOI 10.1007/978-3-319-13057-6_6, © Springer International Publishing Switzerland 2015

The common clinical problems associated with enamel defects are poor esthetics, tooth sensitivity, and increased risk for caries, cusp fracture, tooth wear, and erosion. The management of patients with enamel defects should be focused on early diagnosis, improvement of esthetics, and restoration and preservation of the dentition and often requires interdisciplinary teams consisting of general dentists, pediatric dentists, orthodontists, and prosthodontists. Despite major advances in understanding of the etiology of defects of enamel formation, further research is required to help identify the unknown causes of developmental defects of teeth and deepen the understanding of the functions and of genetic and environmental processes and interactions involved.

Introduction

Consisting of over 98 % mineral and less than 2 % organic matrix and water by weight, dental enamel, consisting mainly of hydroxyapatite, is the hardest tissue found in mammals [49]. The formation of enamel occurs over a long period of time and involves complex and highly coordinated biological mechanisms of laying down and processing of a protein matrix to provide an optimum environment for mineralization. There are known to be over 100 environmental conditions associated with developmental defects of enamel and nearly as many known genetic causes. Not surprisingly, oral health care providers are often challenged with trying to diagnose the etiology of and establish an appropriate approach to manage these diverse and often complex conditions. Most of the processes involved in amelogenesis are controlled directly by the ameloblasts, the cells that produce enamel [49]. Among the numerous proteins involved in enamel formation, amelogenin, which helps control the shape and size of the enamel crystals and is produced by the *AMELX* and *AMELY* genes on the X and Y chromosomes, is the most abundant. Another protein, enamelin, produced by the *ENAM* gene, is associated with the enamel crystal growth and lengthening. Mineralization of the enamel matrix is facilitated by the action of enzymes such as enamelysin or matrix metalloproteinase 20 (*MMP20*), which degrades the matrix proteins [53]. Another key proteinase enzyme, kallikrein-4 (*KLK4*), functions to remove the remaining proteins in the matrix during the maturation stage when the hydroxyapatite crystal growth is complete [42]. Upon completion of enamel formation, many of the ameloblasts undergo programmed cell death (apoptosis) [73].

Hereditary defects of enamel development can be inherited as a result of mutations in the genes that code for proteins involved in enamel formation. Hereditary enamel defects can also occur as a feature of syndromes that have manifestations beyond enamel and in some cases will involve tissues sharing common embryologic origins of neuroectodermal mesenchyme with teeth, such as the hair, teeth, and nails [16]. The aim of this chapter is to review the etiology and clinical manifestations of inherited defects of enamel development and the current treatment approaches to these defects. This chapter will focus on the diagnosis and management of the diverse conditions affecting dental enamel, namely, amelogenesis imperfecta (AI), and medical conditions that feature enamel defects as a prominent part of the syndrome, such as epidermolysis bullosa and tricho-dento-osseous syndrome. While it is not within the scope of this chapter to cover the hundreds of conditions that affect enamel, we provide a framework that oral health care providers can use to diagnose and manage enamel defects.

Amelogenesis Imperfecta

A broad group of genomic disorders that affect the structure and appearance of dental enamel is known as amelogenesis imperfecta (AI). AI has been reported to occur at prevalence rates of approximately 1:14,000 to 1:700 [5, 81]. Based on clinical phenotype, AI has been traditionally classified into hypoplastic, hypocalcified (hypomineralized), or hypomaturation types depending on the stage of enamel formation that is affected by the genetic defect [81]. The hypoplastic phenotypes have a deficient quantity of enamel and usually result from abnormalities of proteins that form or degrade the enamel matrix. They are often characterized by thin enamel, surface pitting, or grooving (Fig. 6.1). In contrast, the hypocalcified phenotypes have defects in initial crystallite formation and defective crystal growth, while the hypomaturation types show defects in the final growth of the enamel crystals (Figs. 6.2, 6.3, and 6.4). The hypocalcified AI phenotypes are associated with mutations in genes coding for proteins involved in hydroxyapatite formation, growth, and mineralization and are characterized by soft, opaque, and discolored enamel that fractures easily.

Genotypes and Phenotypes of Amelogenesis Imperfecta

Recent advances in molecular genetics and biochemistry have made it possible to subtype the AI phenotypes based on the type of genetic mutation. The AI mutations and proteins associated

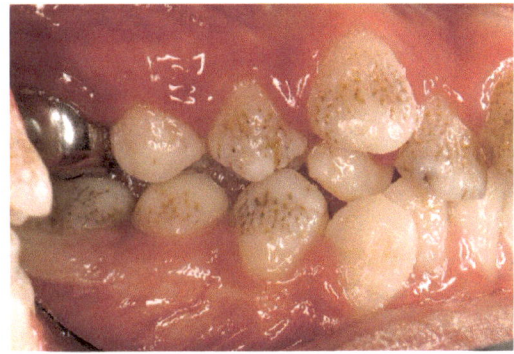

Fig. 6.1 Photograph of the teeth of a 13-year-old boy with hypoplastic AI showing pitted enamel surfaces

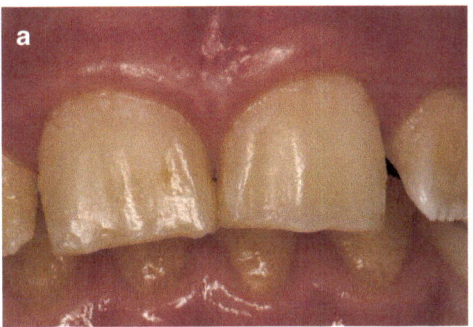
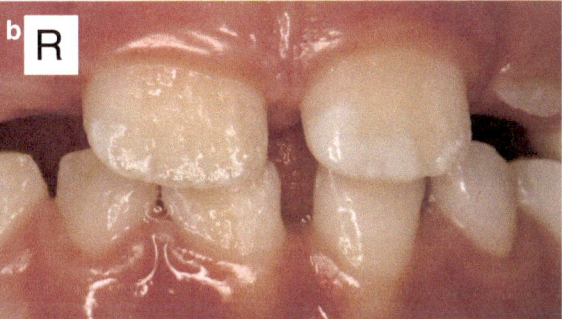

Fig. 6.2 (**a**) Photographs of the maxillary incisors of a boy from a family with X-linked amelogenesis imperfecta showing minimal enamel present. (**b**) Incisors of the sister of the boy in (a) showing pits, irregular ridges of normal enamel, and areas of absent enamel. These features are more noticeable on the right-side incisor

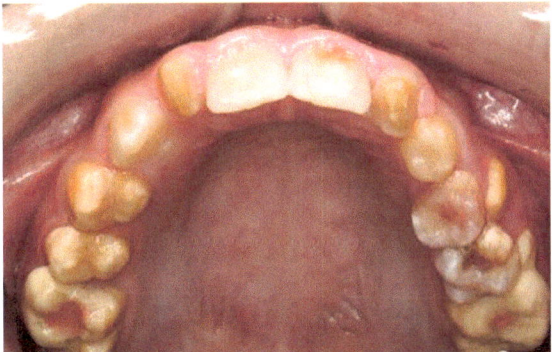
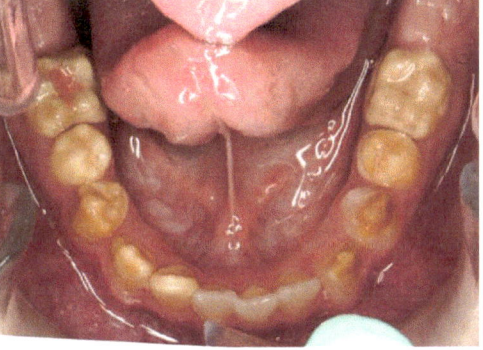

Fig. 6.3 Photographs showing the maxillary and mandibular teeth of an 11-year-old boy with hypocalcified AI

with some of the hypoplastic, hypocalcified, and hypomaturation phenotypes and their modes of inheritance are shown in Tables 6.1 and 6.2, while the OMIM designations and genes involved in some AI conditions are shown in Table 6.3. To date, only approximately half of all AI phenotypes are thought to be caused by mutations in known genes that affect enamel formation, namely, *AMEL*, *ENAM*, *FAM83H*, *KLK4*, *MMP20*, *WDR72*, and *C4ORF26*, while the

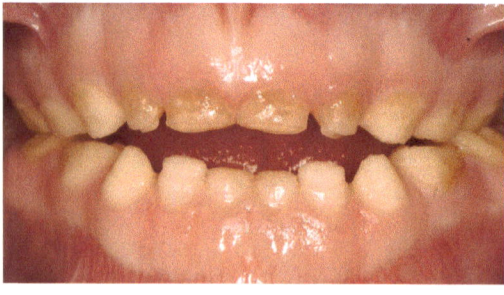

Fig. 6.4 Photographs of a 5-year-old boy's primary dentition that is affected by hypomaturation type of AI showing anterior open bite

genetic changes involved in the other half of AI phenotypes are currently unknown [6, 71, 91].

Mutations in the gene coding for the enamel protein *ENAM* have been reported for two distinct types of AI that are mostly transmitted in an autosomal dominant (AD) manner [28, 31] where the inheritance rate of AI from an affected parent is 1:2 regardless of gender. In addition, a few families with *ENAM* mutations have reported autosomal recessive (AR) transmission [21, 51] where the rate of inheriting AI from two carrier parents is 1:4 regardless of gender (Table 6.1). *ENAM* mutations are associated with hypoplastic phenotypes with the enamel defects presenting as generalized thin or pitted enamel [89]. Some *ENAM* mutations, e.g., in p.K53X [46], are associated with localized defects, most likely from haploinsufficiency (reduced enamel production due to decreased amounts of enamelin that is being produced from the one normal allele). Other types of *ENAM* mutations, e.g., p. N197fsX277 [28], may result in thin or absent enamel, probably as a result of production of

Table 6.1 Phenotypes and genotypes of hypoplastic types of amelogenesis imperfecta

Phenotype	Inheritance	AI mutation	Protein	Authors
Hypoplastic – smooth	AD	ENAM	p.A158Q178del	Rajpar et al. (2001) [57]
Hypoplastic – thin	AD	ENAM	p.N197fsX277	Kida et al. (2002) [28]
Hypoplastic	AD	ENAM	p.M71_Q157del	Kim et al. (2005) [31]
Hypoplastic – localized	AD	ENAM	p.K53X	Mardh et al. (2002) [46]
Hypoplastic – localized	AD	ENAM	p.422fsX277	Hart et al. (2003) [21]
Hypoplastic – localized	AD	ENAM	p.S246X	Ozdemir et al. (2005) [51, 52]
Hypoplastic – smooth, thin	AR	ENAM	p.V340_M341insSQYQYCV	Ozdemir et al. (2005) [51, 52]
Hypoplastic – smooth, thin	AR	ENAM	p.P422fsX448	Hart et al. (2003) [21]
Hypoplastic – smooth	X-linked	AMEL	p.15_a8delinsT	Lagerstrom-Fermer et al. (1991) [38]
Hypoplastic – smooth	X-linked	AMEL	p.W4X	Sekiguchi et al. (2001) [62]
Hypoplastic – smooth	X-linked	AMEL	p.MIT	Kim et al. (2004) [30]
Hypoplastic – smooth	X-linked	AMEL	p.W45	Kim et al. (2004) [30]
Hypoplastic – smooth	X-linked	AMEL	p.E191X	Lench and Winter (1995) [41]
Hypoplastic – smooth	X-linked	AMEL	p.P158fsX187	Lench and Winter (1995) [41]
Hypoplastic – smooth	X-linked	AMEL	p.L181fsX187	Kindelan et al. (2000) [33]
Hypoplastic – smooth	X-linked	AMEL	p.Y147fsX187	Green et al. (2002) [19]
Hypoplastic – smooth	X-linked	AMEL	p.H129fsX187	Sekiguchi et al. (2001) [62]
Hypoplastic – smooth	X-linked	AMEL	p.P52R	Kida et al. (2007) [29]
Hypoplastic – smooth	X-linked	AMEL	pT511	Lench and Winter (1995) [41]

Table 6.2 Phenotypes and genotypes of hypocalcified and hypomaturation types of amelogenesis imperfecta

Phenotype	Inheritance	AI mutation	Protein	Authors
Hypomaturation/hypoplastic	X-linked	AMEL	p.18del	Lagerstrom et al. (1991) [37]
Hypomaturation/hypoplastic	X-linked	AMEL	p.H77L	Hart et al. (2003) [21]
Hypomaturation	X-linked	AMEL	p.P701	Collier et al. (1997) [10]
Hypomaturation	AR	MMP20	p.1319fs338X	Kim et al. (2005) [31]
Hypomaturation	AR	MMP20	p.H226Q	Ozdemir et al. (2005) [51, 52]
Hypomaturation	AR	MMP20	p.W34X	Papagerakis et al. (2008) [53]
Hypomaturation	AR	WDR72	p.Ser783X	El-Sayed et al. (2009) [13]
Hypomaturation	AR	WDR72	p.S489fs498	Wright et al. (2011) [91]
Hypomaturation	AR	WDR72	p.Lys333X	Kuechler et al. (2012) [35]
Hypomaturation	AR	KLK4	p.W153X	Hart et al. (2004) [22]
Hypocalcified	AD	FAM83H	p.S287X	Wright et al. (2009) [88]
Hypocalcified	AD	FAM83H	p.Q470X	Wright et al. (2009) [88]
Hypocalcified	AD	FAM83H	p.Q456X	Hart et al. (2009) [23]
Hypocalcified	AD	FAM83H	p.L308fsX323	Wright et al. (2009) [88]
Hypocalcified	AD	FAM83H	p.W460X	Lee et al. (2008) [39]
Hypocalcified	AD	FAM83H	p.Q677X	Lee et al. (2008) [39]
Hypocalcified – localized	AD	FAM83H	p.L625fsX703	Wright et al. (2009) [88]
Hypocalcified – localized	AD	FAM83H	p.E694X	Wright et al. (2009) [88]

Table 6.3 Hereditary conditions with enamel defects – OMIM designations and genes

Amelogenesis imperfecta	Gene/locus	Enamel phenotype	Mode of inheritance
# 301200. Amelogenesis imperfecta, type IE; AI1E	*AMELX*	Hypoplasia/hypomaturation depending on mutation and protein effect	X-linked
% 301201. Amelogenesis imperfecta, hypoplastic/hypomaturation, X-linked 2	*Xq22-q28*	Hypoplastic and/or hypomaturation	X-linked
#104500. Amelogenesis imperfecta, type IB; AI1B	*ENAM*	Localized hypoplastic/generalized hypoplastic	Autosomal dominant
#204650. Amelogenesis imperfecta, type IC; AI1C	*ENAM*	Generalized hypoplastic	Autosomal dominant
#204700. Amelogenesis imperfecta, hypomaturation type, IIA1; AI2A1	*KLK4*	Normal enamel thickness – hypomineralized orange-brown color	Autosomal recessive
#612529. Amelogenesis imperfecta, hypomaturation type, IIA2; AI2A2	*MMP20*	Normal enamel thickness – hypomineralized orange-brown color	Autosomal recessive
#130900. Amelogenesis imperfecta, type III; AI3	*FAM83H*	Localized or generalized hypomineralized enamel	Autosomal recessive
#613211. Amelogenesis imperfecta, hypomaturation type, IIA3; AI2A3	*WDR72*	Hypomaturation – creamier/opaque enamel upon eruption. Discoloration and loss of tissue post-eruption	Autosomal recessive
#104510. Amelogenesis imperfecta, type IV; AI4	*DLX3*	TDO – thin pitted hypoplastic	Autosomal dominant
# 614253. Amelogenesis imperfecta and gingival fibromatosis syndrome; AIGFS	*FAM20A*	Generalized hypoplastic and failure of tooth eruption, gingival hypertrophy	Autosomal recessive
%104530. Amelogenesis imperfecta, hypoplastic type	???	Hypoplastic – failure to erupt and calcification of pulp. 6 different forms	?
#614832. Amelogenesis imperfecta, hypomaturation, IIA4; AI2A4	*C4ORF26*	Hypomaturation AI	Autosomal recessive

abnormal proteins that are nonfunctional for enamel formation.

The *AMELX* gene encodes for the enamel protein amelogenin which has key roles, which are as yet not fully understood, in the enamel extracellular matrix that undergoes mineralization [72]. As approximately 90 % of human amelogenin is expressed from the *AMELX* gene, and only 10 % from the *AMELY* gene, inheritance of most *AMEL* mutations, is X-linked and is characterized by males typically having a more severe phenotype compared with females [83]. The rate of inheriting the X-linked gene is 1:2 for both male and female children of an affected mother and normal father. For children of an affected father and normal mother, the inheritance rate is 1:2 for female children and none of the male children will inherit the gene. Females with the *AMELX* gene mutations typically show the Lyonization effect where partial X-chromosome inactivation in the ameloblasts results in alternating vertical bands of normal and abnormal enamel [82, 83]. In contrast, affected males usually show a generalized and more severe enamel phenotype compared with females as they are only producing the abnormal protein from the abnormal *AMELX* gene (Fig. 6.2).

Mutations of the *AMELX* gene result in phenotypes that have been reported as hypoplastic or hypomaturation phenotypes (Tables 6.1 and 6.2). Generalized thin hypoplastic AI phenotypes can result from *AMELX* mutations in the C-terminus-coding regions as well as from abnormalities in the formation of signal peptides [38, 39, 61]. In contrast, enamel hypomaturation phenotypes are associated with mutations in the N-terminus-coding region of *AMELX* [20, 37], while mutations in exons 6 and 5 cause a combined hypomaturation-hypoplastic phenotype [2, 29, 40].

Mutations in the *FAM83H* gene result in autosomal dominant hypocalcified AI that is thought to be the most common form of AI in the USA [88]. Although the role of *FAM83H* in other tissues is unclear, the fact that all *FAM83H* mutations reported to date are associated with enamel changes points to the significance of *FAM83H* in enamel formation. Individuals with *FAM83H* mutations show weak, yellow brown discoloration

of the enamel with severely reduced mineral and increased protein content which contrasts with that of hypomaturation AI in being not proline rich [88]. The generalized types of hypocalcified AI affecting the entire crowns result from *FAM83H* mutations that are usually associated with nonfunctional proteins (e.g., p.Q677X). In contrast, the localized types which are caused by mutations associated with less dysfunctional proteins (e.g., p.E694X) result in enamel changes that are seen mainly in the cervical parts of the crowns [88].

Mutations in the genes coding for the proteinases kallikrein-4 (*KLK4*) and metalloproteinase *MMP20* cause hypomaturation phenotypes and are inherited as autosomal recessive traits [42, 86]. The enamel is hypomineralized with a high protein content although the thickness is normal. Kallikrein-4 (*KLK4*) codes for a proteinase that removes remaining proteins during the maturation phase to allow for optimal crystal growth and mineralization [86]. *MMP20* metalloproteinase is required for cleaving amelogenin and ameloblastin during the secretory stage of enamel formation. Multiple allelic mutations in *MMP20* have been identified [18, 32, 52, 53], and the resulting phenotypes are different from the autosomal recessive pigmented hypomaturation AI that is caused by the *C4ORF26* gene mutations. Another group of mutations associated with autosomal recessive hypocalcified or hypomaturation types of AI is found in mutations of the gene *WDR72* that codes for an intracellular protein thought to have mediatory functions between proteins [17, 85].

Other Abnormalities Associated with Amelogenesis Imperfecta

Other oral conditions are encountered in patients with AI more frequently compared to the general population. The most well known of these is skeletal open bites which occur commonly with the hypomaturation and hypocalcified phenotypes (Fig. 6.4) [9, 25, 54]. The etiology of skeletal open bites in AI is unclear, but has been speculated to be associated with effects of the genetic changes in other tissues. It is possible that anterior open bites may also result from abnormal jaw posturing or changes in bite force due to severe dental sensitivity of the AI teeth [9]. Other abnormalities that have been associated with AI include taurodontism, eruption delay/failure, hypercementosis, pulp calcifications [44], impaction of teeth, and follicular cysts [9, 65, 80].

Other Hereditary Conditions with Enamel Defects

Molecular defects can alter enamel development by a variety of mechanisms and there are thousands of genes expressed by ameloblasts supporting their activities toward enamel development. Genetic alterations can exert a direct effect through gene expression by the enamel-forming cells (e.g., ameloblasts secrete an abnormal matrix such as in AI) or by secondary effects where the gene may not be dysfunctional or expressed by the ameloblast (e.g., underlying mesenchymal cells affected or systemic metabolic alteration). Genetic mutations can have a direct effect on the oral epithelium, thereby altering the differentiation or function of the ameloblasts or adjacent supporting cells (e.g., stratum intermedium). For example, junctional epidermolysis bullosa (OMIM 226700, 226650) is associated with enamel hypoplasia secondary to abnormal laminin 5 formation that is critical for cell attachment [1, 87]. Most hereditary conditions affecting enamel formation result in a hypoplastic enamel phenotype. For example, junctional epidermolysis bullosa (JEB) caused by alteration of laminin 5 has a thin and/or pitted enamel phenotype. Because laminin 5 also is a critical component of the epidermal-dermal junction, skin fragility is a hallmark feature of JEB. Depending on the severity of skin fragility, the oral health management of individuals with JEB can be very challenging.

Other conditions such as tricho-dento-osseous syndrome (TDO – OMIM # 190320) that is caused by mutations in the transcription factor *DLX3* also have a thin and/or pitted enamel phenotype. Affected individuals are almost always born with kinky-curly hair (half of them lose this characteristic by childhood) and dense cranial and skeletal bone that becomes apparent on radiographs during childhood [90]. There is marked variability in affected individuals despite almost all of the cases having the same genetic mutation in the *DLX3* gene. Taurodontism and large pulp chambers with thin dentin are a common feature of this condition and help delineate it from AI. The propensity for developing pulp necrosis and having abscess formation appears to stem from the combination of thin enamel, large pulps, and thin dentin that allow microexposure of the dental pulp and bacterial invasion. Placing resin copings or crowns to help prevent pulp exposure can be beneficial in the primary and developing permanent dentition in more severely affected individuals.

There are numerous forms of ectodermal dysplasias that can have significant enamel defects such as Goltz syndrome (also called focal dermal hypoplasia – OMIM # 305600) and ectrodactyly, ectodermal dysplasia, and cleft lip/palate syndrome (OMIM # 604292) to name just a couple. While most syndromes are associated with a hypoplastic enamel phenotype, the severity of the enamel defect varies markedly, and there can be many associated features such as hypodontia and facial clefting as examples. Therefore, the management of each of these conditions will be different depending on the nature of the enamel defects (e.g., hypoplastic and/or hypomineralized) and the presence of associated oral and systemic conditions.

Management of Patients with Hereditary Defects of Enamel Development

Clinical problems commonly experienced by many patients affected with developmental defects of enamel, regardless of whether they are associated with AI or a syndrome, are compromised esthetics, dental sensitivity, tooth wear, and increased risk for caries and calculus formation [47, 64]. Management of enamel defects will be predicated on understanding and accounting for the associated oral and systemic manifestations and potential need for special medical management (e.g., treatment of severe EB conditions). The severity of the enamel defects and associated problems varies depending on the specific condition. For example, with the AI conditions the hypocalcified and hypomaturation variants have more severe signs and symptoms compared with the hypoplastic types. The aims of dental treatment are to reduce dental sensitivity, improve esthetics, restore masticatory function, and prevent deterioration of the dentition from caries, fracture, tooth wear, and erosion. Early diagnosis and preventive care are essential for effective preservation of the dentition. Clinicians should also be alert to the fact that psychological distress and low self-esteem are prevalent among AI children, particularly those with the more severe types, presumably from the reduced quality of life associated with poor esthetics and tooth sensitivity [8, 24]. Children who have a family history of AI or medical syndromes that are commonly associated with defects of enamel development such as epidermolysis bullosa should be examined as soon as the primary and permanent teeth emerge [66]. Referral to specialist pediatric dentists, pediatricians, and geneticists for definitive diagnosis, genetic testing, and counseling may be required.

In clinical practice, management of patients with developmental enamel defects may be considered in a few age-related phases: 1–6 years old (primary dentition or initial phase), 6–12 years old (early permanent dentition or transitional phase), and teenagers and adults (full permanent dentition). Treatment planning is likely to be complex and, for children and adolescents, usually involves interdisciplinary specialists including general dental practitioners, specialist pediatric dentists, and orthodontists. A prosthodontist may need to be consulted when the children reach adulthood to manage the complex prosthodontic treatment that is usually required. The preservation of tooth structure should be a central strategy for all patients with enamel defects, and dental management should aim at preventing caries, maintaining good gingival health, and restoring the teeth with minimally invasive treatment options. Maintaining the dentition and alveolar bone is critics so that future implants or prostheses will have optimal bony support.

Preventive Care

For all children with defects of enamel development, the restorative, prosthetic, and orthodontic treatments should be supported by an aggressive program of preventive care. Oral hygiene instruction, diet counseling, topical fluoride therapy, and frequent periodic examinations should be instituted immediately after diagnosis. Preventive care is crucial as children's enamel defects such as AI are at high risk for caries and periodontal disease due to the presence of rough defective enamel surfaces that often extend subgingivally and render oral hygiene difficult. In addition, many children, particularly those with hypocalcified and hypomaturation AI phenotypes, have a higher tendency for calculus formation, probably due to changes on the enamel surfaces, saliva, or plaque microbial flora [84]. Gingival overgrowth may occur as an exaggerated response to retained bacterial plaque and mechanical irritation of abnormal enamel that may further compromise esthetics [45]. As AI children often have difficulties with oral hygiene due to tooth sensitivity, toothbrushing and flossing techniques should be taught to the parents and child and reinforced frequently. Short recalls for professional scaling and cleaning are recommended for children who are unable to perform oral hygiene thoroughly [47]. Antibacterial mouth rinses or gels such as chlorhexidine may help some patients, particularly adolescents, achieve optimum gingival health before and after restorative work and after periodontal surgery [84].

Preventive agents for caries prevention for children with AI or other enamel defects include neutral sodium fluoride gels or varnishes applied professionally three or six times monthly [59]. Daily or weekly neutral sodium fluoride mouth rinses may be prescribed for children older than 6 years of age who are capable of spitting out the mouth rinse. Calcium- and phosphate-rich products such as casein phosphopeptide amorphous calcium phosphate creams (CPP-ACP) have been recommended as they encourage remineralization [7, 58, 92]. However, to date, there are no controlled clinical studies showing that CPP-ACP is effective for managing teeth with AI or other forms of hypomineralized enamel (e.g., molar-incisor hypomineralization).

Anterior Teeth Restorations

Although a recent Cochrane review concluded that due to the absence of randomized controlled trials, there is no evidence as to which is the best restorative treatment for AI [11], there are several reports of case series and individual patients that provide useful information regarding treatment options for AI children, adolescents, and adults.

In patients with AI, the anterior teeth often need to be restored to improve esthetics and protect them from caries and erosion [64]. In young children and adolescents with the hypoplastic AI phenotypes where there is sufficient enamel, these aims would be achievable with acid-etched composite resins bonded directly to the teeth. However, in males with X-linked AI where minimal enamel is present or the smooth hypoplastic AI phenotypes where the etching effect on the enamel surface is inadequate, composite resins are less likely to be successful unless combined with other approaches such as obtaining mechanical retention and the use of dentin-bonding resins [67].

Composite resins for anterior teeth affected with AI or other enamel defects frequently should envelope the entire crown wherever possible to provide maximum retention, protection, and esthetics. In cases of deep overbite, it may be necessary to limit the placement of composite resins to the facial aspects. Enamel discolorations which are frequently encountered in the hypocalcified and hypomaturation AI phenotypes may be removed using microabrasion, employing an acidic slurry containing 18 % hydrochloric acid and pumice [50, 56]. A coating of composite resin is usually recommended after removal of the discolorations to protect the enamel surface and prevent recurrence of the stains. Composite resins containing opaque fillers may also be applied to mask the discolorations. If the composite resins are inserted prior to full eruption of the permanent anterior teeth, the existing resto-

rations may be readily modified as the teeth erupt by adding more material to the gingival margins. To improve the bonding of the composite resins to enamel that is poorly mineralized, pretreatment of the surface with 5 % hypochlorite solution has been proposed as a method to remove excess proteins and improve bond strength [60, 74]. Bleaching the affected teeth after mechanical preparation for 60 s also improves coloration and reduces the need in some cases to use an opaque resin restorative material. In some AI-affected teeth that have minimal enamel available for bonding of composite resins, dentin-bonding agents or glass ionomer cements may be used as a dentin-bonding base, on which a composite resin restoration may be placed ("sandwich technique") [48].

Primary anterior teeth affected by AI or other enamel defects may be similarly restored with composite resin veneers and crowns which can be fabricated directly or indirectly [75]. In cases where there is inadequate retention of directly bonded composite resins, the primary anterior teeth may be fitted with stainless-steel crowns that contain composite resin open face inserts or have prefabricated resin facings [69]. Primary anterior teeth can also be restored with crowns made of zirconium that provide excellent esthetics. These crowns are available through multiple vendors and are made for both maxillary and mandibular anterior teeth.

During the early mixed dentition, the height of gingival contour continues to change and the dental pulp chambers are quite large. For these reasons, it is typically preferable to cover the newly erupting permanent incisors with resin after minimal enamel removal. This will allow for improved esthetics and control of sensitivity. As the teeth continue to erupt, new resin can be added to the newly exposed tooth in the gingival area. In the early permanent dentition, once the gingival height is better established (12–18 years), porcelain veneers may be considered if there is sufficient enamel for bonding and the added esthetics is critical at this time [93]. When the patients reach adulthood and the facial, occlusal, and gingival heights are stable, porcelain and other custom-made full crowns may be considered for maximum esthetics [79].

Posterior Teeth Restorations

In mildly affected cases of AI or conditions with a hypoplastic enamel phenotype, small carious lesions on posterior teeth may be successfully restored using conventional, conservative, intracoronal, restorative materials such as amalgams and composite resins in both primary and permanent dentitions. However, if the enamel phenotype involves hypomineralization of the enamel, the teeth are structurally weak and the tooth structure surrounding intracoronal restorations often fractures, resulting in marginal leakage around restorations, recurrent caries, and pulp involvement [64]. The presence of an adhesive bond between the restorative materials and the affected tooth structure may prevent fracture, and materials such as resin-modified glass ionomer cements and polyacid-modified composite resins that can be bonded to the tooth potentially have greater success rates compared to the nonbonding materials. Clinical studies as to the success of bonded versus non-bonded restorations in patients with developmental defects of the dentition are lacking at this time. These materials are thus are often better suited for teeth with hypomineralized or structurally altered enamel over the nonbonding type of intracoronal materials such as amalgams [64].

When the enamel is poorly mineralized such as the hypocalcified and hypomaturation AI phenotypes, the enamel tends to fracture readily in posterior teeth that are subjected to heavy masticatory stresses. Thus molars are often best protected using full-coverage crowns as soon as the teeth are fully erupted. Complete coverage of the teeth with crowns also reduces tooth sensitivity and helps maintain space and crown height [64]. Stainless steel crowns are typically the most suitable full coverage crown in the young permanent dentition as very little tooth structure removal is required and these crowns have an excellent success rate.

Stainless-steel crowns are highly durable restorations for protecting both primary and young permanent molars affected by enamel hypoplasia [34] (Fig. 6.5). If the teeth are relatively intact, the crowns are best inserted using a conservative technique with minimal removal of tooth structure. This method which involves interproximal separation and minimal or no occlusal surface reduction was

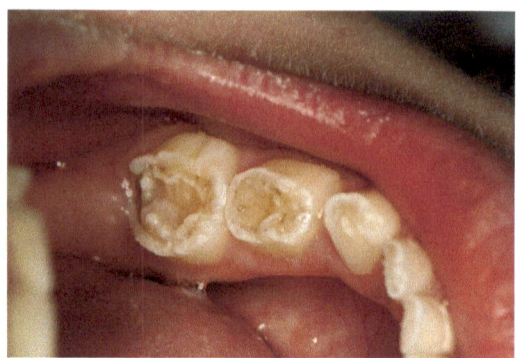

Fig. 6.5 Generalized enamel hypoplasia is evident in the primary dentition of this child affected with junctional epidermolysis bullosa

first introduced for placement of crowns to protect teeth with large pulps to prevent pulp exposures [63, 68]. In this technique, the proximal contacts are opened by applying elastic orthodontic separators a few days prior to crown insertion, and only minimal tooth preparation limited to removal of caries and unsupported enamel is performed [66].

If the insertion of stainless-steel crowns is required for bilateral molar teeth, to avoid discomfort associated with an uneven occlusion, it is recommended that both of either maxillary or mandibular molar crowns be inserted at the first visit, followed by bilateral placement of the opposing crowns at the following visit. In most cases, immediately after insertion of the first set of stainless-steel crowns, the occlusal height is increased by 2–3 mm measured incisally. This change in occlusal height usually returns to normal within 6 weeks in young children and teenagers when the second set of stainless-steel crowns can be inserted.

Esthetic posterior composite resin crowns which are constructed indirectly [55] may be suitable alternatives for molars with hypoplastic or hypomineralized enamel defects, although they lack the strength of stainless-steel crowns and have higher rates of fracture. Full zirconium crowns are also esthetic alternatives for full coverage of primary and permanent molar teeth [70]. However, these crowns are costly and require relatively extensive tooth reduction compared to stainless-steel crowns.

An alternative to full-coverage crowns in the permanent dentition is the precast chrome onlay which protects the occlusal surface. To avoid the necessity for occlusal reduction, the onlays may be inserted supra-occlusally on permanent molars prior to full eruption [26]. Composite resin onlays constructed using indirect techniques have also been proposed for young permanent molars affected by AI [3], although the longevity of these restorations is unclear. In severely affected AI teeth where there is fracture and loss of tooth structure prior to full eruption, glass ionomer cements may be placed as interim restorations until the molar teeth are fully emerged and stainless-steel crowns can be inserted. Glass ionomer cements are particularly useful for teeth affected by AI due to their ability to bond to dentin, fluoride-releasing properties, and the relative ease of insertion [48].

Orthodontic Management of Dentitions Affected by Defects of Enamel Development

Orthodontic treatment for children with AI may be required for general malocclusions as well as conditions that are frequently encountered in AI such as anterior open bites and delayed or non-eruption of the teeth. In addition, in some patients with AI, the excessive interdental spacing associated with thin enamel can be reduced or closed by orthodontic treatment. In severe cases of skeletal open bites, orthognathic surgery may be undertaken in young adults together with orthodontic treatment to achieve an optimal occlusion and facial profile [25, 84].

Orthodontic treatment for AI children and adolescents is associated with increased risks for fracture of the weak enamel due to forces applied during treatment and when removing fixed orthodontic appliances [4]. Repeated bond failures may also prolong orthodontic treatment. Although fixed appliances bonded with acid-etched composite resins may be used for most AI patients, achieving adequate bond strengths may be problematic, particularly in the phenotypes with absent or smooth, thin hypoplastic enamel [67]. Glass ionomer cements may be more suitable compared to composite resin cements for teeth in AI phenotypes with absent enamel due to their ability to bond to

dentine and fluoride-releasing properties which help to prevent enamel demineralization [59].

Plastic brackets can substitute for metal brackets for AI patients as they can be debonded relatively easily with a hand instrument with less risk of damage to the enamel surface. Traditional banded appliances may also be considered if brackets cannot be bonded sufficiently. Additionally, preformed stainless-steel crowns with welded tubes or brackets may be another option if there is insufficient crown height for bracket attachment [4].

Molar-Incisor Hypomineralization

Molar-incisor hypomineralization (MIH) is a developmental defect that primarily affects the enamel of the first permanent molars and incisors. This condition has been described using a variety of terms (e.g., cheese molars, idiopathic hypomineralization of enamel) [76] with the term molar-incisor hypomineralization being accepted by leaders in the field in 2000 [77]. The clinical characteristics are variable between cases and teeth even in the same individual. The hypomineralized enamel defects vary from small, well-demarcated areas of color change to extensive hypomineralization involving the entire dental crown. Affected teeth form with a normal thickness of enamel and the abnormal areas of enamel have a decreased mineral content and increased protein and water content. Discoloration of the affected enamel results from the decreased mineral content and increased protein and water content of enamel that change its optical character [14]. Color changes vary from white opaque lesions to a creamy yellow or brown. The more severely affected the enamel (less mineral), the more likely it is to fracture under function and to cause dental hypersensitivity (Fig. 6.6). The degree of hypersensitivity associated with these defects varies but can be quite pronounced. Hypersensitivity and difficulty anesthetizing the affected molars can add to the challenge of treating individuals with MIH [78].

The prevalence of MIH ranges from about 3–40 %, depending on the population studied, making it a common enamel defect and one that will

Fig. 6.6 Taurodontism, thin enamel, impacted teeth and pulpal involvement are commonly seen in TDO as observed in this affected individuals panoramic radiograph

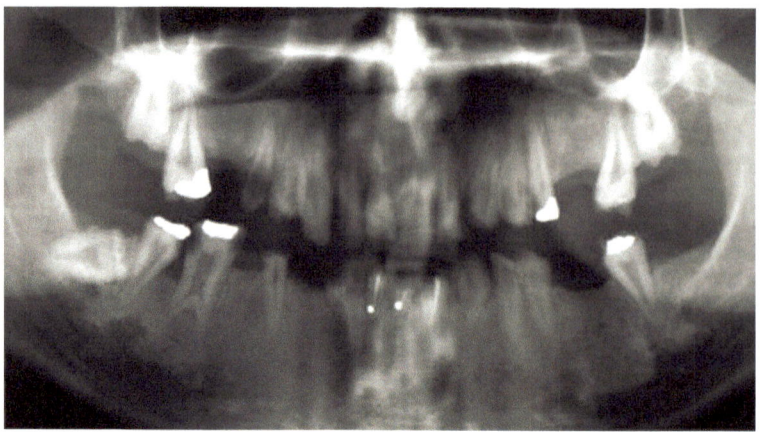

challenge clinicians on a regular basis [27]. The MIH-affected first permanent molar is highly likely to develop dental caries and frequently are associated with hypersensitivity. Having enamel hypomineralization in the primary dentition increases the likelihood that the individual will have MIH in the permanent dentition [12]. Numerous environmental stressors and childhood illnesses have been associated with MIH with most of these stressors occurring in the first year of life [15]. Studies of multiple siblings affected with MIH and a recent study identifying a genetic loci associated with MIH suggest that the etiology of this condition may be complex and involves both environmental stressors and a genetic predisposition [36].

Management of MIH

Treatment approaches for MIH will vary and should be based on the severity, extent, and distribution of the enamel defects. As discussed above, for AI and syndrome-associated enamel defects, the treatment goals are to prevent the tooth from developing dental caries, to help prevent or reduce enamel loss, to restore form and function when there is enamel loss, and to address esthetic issues when the incisors are involved [43, 78]. Management should consist of a combination of preventive and, in moderate to severe cases of MIH where enamel is lost, restorative approaches. Preventive approaches primarily consist of

fluorides and sealant materials. Restorative approaches range from glass ionomers or resins to full-coverage crowns depending on the extent of the lesions, dental hypersensitivity, ability to achieve moisture control, and patient age. In severe cases, extraction can be an ideal approach and should be considered after comprehensive evaluation of the potential ramifications that extraction may have on the occlusion and long-term growth and development (e.g., whether the second or third permanent molars are present). In molars that are discolored but have little or no enamel loss, they often are best managed conservatively with sealants or resin restorations. Deproteinization with sodium hypochlorite (NaOCl) can help achieve a more normal color of enamel, and there is evidence that it can aid in the bonding of resins by removing proteins and allowing better penetration of the resin into the etched enamel. Deproteinization can be accomplished by treating the enamel for 60 s with 5 % NaOCl and then rinsing and proceeding with etching as for conventional sealant or resin placement. This approach may also be helpful for treating forms of AI that are associated with increased enamel protein content (i.e., hypocalcified and hypomaturation AI types). Molars severely affected with MIH that are associated with marked enamel loss and severe sensitivity are often best managed initially with glass ionomers. These materials allow placement of a restoration that will adhere to the tooth structure

Table 6.4 Management of molar-incisor hypomineralization

	Mild	Moderate	Severe
Molars	Desensitizing toothpaste	Fluoride varnish	Glass ionomer coverage
	Fluoride varnish	Sealants	Interim resins
	Sealants	Glass ionomer/resin restorations	Stainless-steel crowns
			Extraction
Incisors	No treatment	Bleach/seal	Bleach/seal
	Resin perfusion	Resin perfusion	Resin perfusion
		Microabrasion	Microabrasion
		Resin restorations	Resin restorations
			Veneers

without optimal moisture control and is very effective for reducing dental sensitivity. This approach allows the patient to maintain the molars until a more definitive approach can be implemented. Incisor esthetics also will be managed by a variety of approaches depending on the location, extent, and severity of the enamel defects (Table 6.4). Treatment approaches for incisors vary from bleaching to resin restorations to veneers. Crowns on MIH-affected incisors are not typically necessary as most incisor involvement is not associated with the marked enamel loss or sensitivity to the same degree as molars.

Conclusions

The etiologies of enamel defects are extremely diverse and the clinician must delineate between a myriad of genetic and environmental causes to obtain a diagnosis. Understanding the nature of the enamel defect (hypoplastic versus hypomineralized) will aid the clinician in selecting treatment approaches and materials that are most likely to produce a successful outcome. The molecular defects causing these conditions are becoming rapidly identified, providing clinicians with objective diagnostic tests to help establish specific diagnoses. Similarly, the environmental conditions that influence the processes involved in enamel formation are also becoming better understood. In the future better technology and materials may provide additional opportunities to help prevent and manage developmental defects of enamel.

References

1. Aberdam D, Aguzzi A, Baudoin C, Galliano M-F, Ortonne J-P, Meneguzzi G. Developmental expression of nicein adhesion protein (laminin-5) subunits suggests multiple morphogenic roles. Cell Adhes Commun. 1994;2:115–29.
2. Aldred MJ, Crawford PJ, Roberts E, Thomas NS. Identification of a nonsense mutation in the amelogenin gene (AMELX) in a family with X-linked amelogenesis imperfecta (AIH1). Hum Genet. 1992;90:413–6.
3. Ardu S, Duc O, Krejci I, Perroud R. Amelogenesis imperfecta: a conservative and progressive adhesive treatment concept. Oper Dent. 2013;38:235–41.
4. Arkutu N, Gadhia K, Mcdonald S, Malik K, Currie L. Amelogenesis imperfecta: the orthodontic perspective. Br Dent J. 2012;212:485–9.
5. Bäckman B, Holm AK. Amelogenesis imperfecta: prevalence and incidence in a northern Swedish county. Community Dent Oral Epidemiol. 1986;14:43–7.
6. Chan HC, Estrella NMRP, Milkovich RN, Kim JW, Simmer JP, Hu JCC. Target gene analyses of 39 amelogenesis imperfecta kindreds. Eur J Oral Sci. 2011;119 Suppl 1:311–23.
7. Cochrane NJ, Saranathan S, Cai F, Cross KJ, Reynolds EC. Enamel subsurface lesion remineralisation with casein phosphopeptide stabilised solutions of calcium, phosphate and fluoride. Caries Res. 2008;42:88–97.
8. Coffield KD, Phillips C, Brady M, Roberts MW, Strauss RP, Wright JT. The psychosocial impact of developmental dental defects in people with hereditary amelogenesis imperfecta. J Am Dent Assoc. 2005;136:620–30.
9. Collins MA, Mauriello SM, Tyndall DA, Wright JT. Dental anomalies associated with amelogenesis imperfecta: a radiographic assessment. Oral Surg Oral Med Oral Pathol Oral Radiol Endod. 1999;88:358–64.

10. Collier PM, Sauk JJ, Rosenbloom SJ, Yuan ZA, Gibson CW. An amelogenin gene defect associated with human X-linked amelogenesis imperfecta. Arch Oral Biol. 1997;42:235–42.

11. Dashash M, Yeung CA, Jamous I, Blinkhorn A. Interventions for the restorative care of amelogenesis imperfecta in children and adolescents. Cochrane Database Syst Rev. 2013;6:CD007157.

12. Elfrink ME, ten Cate JM, Jaddoe VW, Hofman A, Moll HA, Veerkamp JS. Deciduous molar hypomineralization and molar incisor hypomineralization. J Dent Res. 2012;91:551–5.

13. El-Sayed W, Parry DA, Shore RC, Ahmed M, Jafri H, Rashid Y, Al-Bahlani S, Al Harasi S, Kirkham J, Inglehearn CF, Mighell JA. Mutations in the beta propeller WDR72 cause autosomal-recessive hypomaturation amelogenesis imperfecta. Am J Hum Genet. 2009;85:699–705.

14. Fagrell T. Molar incisor hypomineralization. Morphological and chemical aspects, onset and possible etiological factors. Swed Dent J Suppl. 2011;5:11–83.

15. Fagrell TG, Salmon P, Melin L, Noren JG. Onset of molar incisor hypomineralization (MIH). Swed Dent J. 2013;37:61–70.

16. Freiman A, Borsuk D, Barankin B, Sperber GH, Krafchik B. Dental manifestations of dermatologic conditions. J Am Acad Dermatol. 2009;60:289–98.

17. Gadhia K, Mcdonald S, Arkutu N, Malik K. Amelogenesis imperfecta: an introduction. Br Dent J. 2012;212:377–9.

18. Gasse B, Karayigit E, Mathieu E, Jung S, Garret A, Huckert M, Morkmued S, Schneider C, Vidal L, Hemmerle J, Sire JY, Bloch-Zupan A. Homozygous and compound heterozygous MMP20 mutations in amelogenesis imperfecta. J Dent Res. 2013;92:598–603.

19. Greene SR, Yuan ZA, Wright JT, Amjad H, Abrams WR, Buchanan JA, Trachtenberg DI, Gibson CW. A new frameshift mutation encoding a truncated amelogenin leads to X-linked amelogenesis imperfecta. Arch Oral Biol. 2002;47:211–7.

20. Hart PS, Aldred MJ, Crawford PJM, Wright NJ, Hart TC, Wright JT. Amelogenesis imperfecta phenotype – genotype correlations with two amelogenin gene mutations. Arch Oral Biol. 2002;47:261–5.

21. Hart T, Hart P, Gorry M, Michalec M, Ryu O, Uygur C, Ozdemir D, Firatli S, Aren G, Firatli E. Novel ENAM mutation responsible for autosomal recessive amelogenesis imperfecta and localised enamel defects. J Med Genet. 2003;40:900–6.

22. Hart PS, Hart TC, Michalec MD, Ryu OH, Simmons D, Hong S, Wright JT. Mutation in kallikrein 4 causes autosomal recessive hypomaturation amelogenesis imperfecta. J Med Genet. 2004;41:545–9.

23. Hart PS, Becerik S, Cogulu D, Emingil G, Ozdemir-Ozenen D, Han ST, Sulima PP, Firatli E, Hart TC. Novel FAM83H mutations in Turkish families with autosomal dominant hypocalcified amelogenesis imperfecta. Clin Genet. 2009;75:401–4.

24. Hashem A, Kelly A, O'Connell B, O'Sullivan M. Impact of moderate and severe hypodontia and amelogenesis imperfecta on quality of life and self-esteem of adult patients. J Dent. 2013;41:689.

25. Hoppenreijs TJM, Voorsmit RACA, Freihofer HPM. Open bite deformity in amelogenesis imperfecta part 1: an analysis of contributory factors and implications for treatment. J Cranio-Maxillofac Surg. 1998;26:260–6.

26. Hunter L, Stone D. Supraoccluding cobalt-chrome onlays in the management of amelogenesis imperfecta in children: a 2-year case report. Quintessence Int. 1997;28:15–9.

27. Jalevik B. Prevalence and diagnosis of Molar-Incisor-Hypomineralisation (MIH): a systematic review. Eur Arch Paediatr Dent. 2010;11:59–64.

28. Kida M, Ariga T, Shirakawa T, Oguchi H, Sakiyama Y. Autosomal-dominant hypoplastic form of amelogenesis imperfecta caused by an enamelin gene mutation at the exon-intron boundary. J Dent Res. 2002;81:738–42.

29. Kida M, Sakiyama Y, Matsuda A, Takabayashi S, Ochi H, Sekiguchi H, Minamitake S, Ariga T. A novel missense mutation (p.P52R) in amelogenin gene causing X-linked amelogenesis imperfecta. J Dent Res. 2007;86:69–72.

30. Kim J-W, Simmer JP, Hu YY, Lin BP, Boyd C, Wright JT, Yamada CJ, Rayes SK, Feigal RJ, Hu JC. Amelogenin p.M1T and p.W4S mutations underlying hypoplastic X-linked amelogenesis imperfecta. J Dent Res. 2004;83:378–83.

31. Kim J, Seymen F, Lin B, Kiziltan B, Gencay K, Simmer J, Hu J. ENAM mutations in autosomal-dominant amelogenesis imperfecta. J Dent Res. 2005;84:278–82.

32. Kim J, Simmer J, Hart T, Hart P, Ramaswami M, Bartlett J, Hu J. MMP-20 mutation in autosomal recessive pigmented hypomaturation amelogenesis imperfecta. J Med Genet. 2005;42:271–5.

33. Kindelan SA, Brook AH, Gangemi L, Lench N, Wong FS, Fearne J, Jackson Z, Foster G, Stringer BM. Detection of a novel mutation in X-linked amelogenesis imperfecta. J Dent Res. 2000;79:1978–82.

34. Kindelan SA, Day P, Nichol R, Willmott N, Fayle SA. UK national clinical guidelines in paediatric dentistry: stainless steel preformed crowns for primary molars. Int J Paediatr Dent. 2008;18:20–8.

35. Kuechler A, Hentschel J, Kurth I, Stephan B, Prott EC, Schweiger B, Schuster A, Wieczorek D, Ludecke HJ. A novel homozygous WDR72 mutation in two siblings with mmelogenesis imperfecta and mild short stature. Molecular Syndromol. 2012;3:223–9.

36. Kühnisch J, Thiering E, Heitmüller D, Tiesler CM, Grallert H, Heinrich-Weltzien R, Hickel R, Heinrich J, GINI-10 Plus Study Group, LISA-10Plus Study Group. Genome-wide association study (GWAS) for molar-incisor hypomineralization (MIH). Clin Oral Investig. 2014;18:677–82.

37. Lagerstrom M, Dahl N, Nakahori Y, Nakagome Y, Backman B, Landegren U, Pettersson U. A deletion in the amelogenin gene (AMG) causes X-linked amelogenesis imperfecta (AIH1). Genomics. 1991;10:971–5.

38. Lagerstrom-Fermer M, Nilsson M, Backman B, Salido E, Shapiro L, Pettersson U, Landegren U. Amelogenin signal peptide mutation: correlation between mutations in the amelogenin gene (AMGX) and manifestations of X-linked amelogenesis imperfecta. Genomics. 1995;26:159–62.

39. Lee SK, Hu JC, Bartlett JD, Lee KE, Lin BP, Simmer JP, Kim JW. Mutational spectrum of FAM83H: the C-terminal portion is required for tooth enamel calcification. Hum Mutat. 2008;29:E95–9.

40. Lench NJ, Brook AH, Winter GB. SSCP detection of a nonsense mutation in exon 5 of the amelogenin gene (AMGX) causing X-linked amelogenesis imperfecta (AIH1). Hum Mol Genet. 1994;3:827–8.

41. Lench N, Winter G. Characterisation of molecular defects in X-linked amelogenesis imperfecta (AIH1). Hum Mutat. 1995;5:251–9.

42. Lu Y, Papagerakis P, Yamakoshi Y, Hu Jan CC, Bartlett JD, Simmer JP. Functions of KLK4 and MMP-20 in dental enamel formation. Biol Chem. 2008;389:695–700.

43. Lygidakis NA, Wong F, Jalevik B, Vierrou AM, Alaluusua S, Espelid I. Best clinical practice guidance for clinicians dealing with children presenting with Molar-Incisor-Hypomineralisation (MIH): an EAPD policy document. Eur Arch Paediatr Dent. 2010; 11:75–81.

44. Lykogeorgos T, Duncan K, Crawford PJM, Aldred MJ. Unusual manifestations in X-linked amelogenesis imperfecta. Int J Paediatr Dent. 2003;13:356–61.

45. Macedo GO, Tunes RS, Motta AC, Passador-Santos F, Grisi MM, Souza SL, Palioto DB, Taba Jr M, Novaes Jr AB. Amelogenesis imperfecta and unusual gingival hyperplasia. J Periodontol. 2005;76:1563–6.

46. Mardh C, Backman B, Holmgren G, Hu J, Simmer J, Forsman-Semb K. A nonsense mutation in the enamelin gene causes local hypoplastic autosomal dominant amelogenesis imperfecta (AIH2). Hum Mol Genet. 2002;11:1069–74.

47. Markovic D, Petrovic B, Peric T. Case series: clinical findings and oral rehabilitation of patients with amelogenesis imperfecta. Eur Arch Paediatr Dent. 2010;11:201–8.

48. Mount GJ. Longevity in glass-ionomer restorations: review of a successful technique. Quintessence Int. 1997;28:643–50.

49. Nanci A. Enamel: composition, formation, and structure. In: Nanci AE, editor. Ten Cate's oral histology development, structure, and function. St Louis: Mosby; 2008.

50. Nathwani NS, Kelleher M. Minimally destructive management of amelogenesis imperfecta and hypodontia with bleaching and bonding. Dent Update. 2010;37:170–2, 175–6, 179.

51. Ozdemir D, Hart P, Firatli E, Aren G, Ryu O, Hart T. Phenotype of ENAM mutations is dosage-dependent. J Dent Res. 2005;84:1036–41.

52. Ozdemir D, Hart P, Ryu O, Choi S, Ozdemir-Karatas M, Firatli E, Piesco N, Hart T. MMP20 active-site mutation in hypomaturation amelogenesis imperfecta. J Dent Res. 2005;84:1031–5.

53. Papagerakis P, Lin HK, Lee KY, Hu Y, Simmer JP, Bartlett JD, Hu JC. Premature stop codon in MMP20 causing amelogenesis imperfecta. J Dent Res. 2008;87:56–9.

54. Persson M, Sundell S. Facial morphology and open bite deformity in amelogenesis imperfecta: a roentgenocephalometric study. Acta Odontol Scand. 1982;40:135–44.

55. Preissner S, Kostka E, Blunck U. A noninvasive treatment of amelogenesis imperfecta. Quintessence Int. 2013;44:303–5.

56. Price RB, Loney RW, Doyle MG, Moulding MB. An evaluation of a technique to remove stains from teeth using microabrasion. J Am Dent Assoc. 2003;134:1066–71.

57. Rajpar M, Harley K, Laing C, Davies R, Dixon M. Mutation of the gene encoding the enamel-specific protein, enamelin, causes autosomal-dominant amelogenesis imperfecta. Hum Mol Genet. 2001; 10:1673–7.

58. Ranjitkar S, Rodriguez JM, Kaidonis JA, Richards LC, Townsend GC, Bartlett DW. The effect of casein phosphopeptide-amorphous calcium phosphate on erosive enamel and dentine wear by toothbrush abrasion. J Dent. 2009;37:250–4.

59. Sapir S, Shapira J. Clinical solutions for developmental defects of enamel and dentin in children. Pediatr Dent. 2007;29:330–6.

60. Saroglu I, Aras S, Oztas D. Effect of deproteinization on composite bond strength in hypocalcified amelogenesis imperfecta. Oral Dis. 2006;12:305–8.

61. Sekiguchi H, Minaguchi K, Machida Y, Yakushiji M. PCR detection of the human amelogenin gene and its application to the diagnosis of amelogenesis imperfecta. Bull Tokyo Dent Coll. 1998;39: 275–85.

62. Sekiguchi H, Tanakamaru H, Minaguchi K, Machida Y, Yakushiji M. A case of amelogenesis imperfecta of the deciduous and all permanent teeth. Bull Tokyo Dent Coll. 2001;42:45–50.

63. Seow WK. The application of tooth-separation in clinical pedodontics. J Dent Child. 1984;51:428–30.

64. Seow WK. Clinical diagnosis and management strategies of amelogenesis imperfecta variants. Pediatr Dent. 1993;15:384–93.

65. Seow WK. Dental development in amelogenesis imperfecta: a controlled study. Pediatr Dent. 1995;17:26–30.

66. Seow WK. Developmental defects of enamel and dentine: challenges for basic science research and clinical management. Aust Dent J. 2014;59(1 Suppl): 1–12.

67. Seow WK, Amaratunge A. The effects of acid-etching on enamel from different clinical variants of amelogenesis imperfecta: an SEM study. Pediatr Dent. 1998,20:37–42.

68. Seow WK, Latham SC. The spectrum of dental manifestations in vitamin D-resistant rickets: implications for management. Pediatr Dent. 1986;8:245–50.

69. Shah PV, Lee JY, Wright JT. Clinical success and parental satisfaction with anterior preveneered pri-

mary stainless steel crowns. Pediatr Dent. 2004; 26:391–5.

70. Siadat H, Alikhasi M, Mirfazaelian A. Rehabilitation of a patient with amelogenesis imperfecta using all-ceramic crowns: a clinical report. J Prosthet Dent. 2007;98:85–8.

71. Simmer SG, Estrella NMRP, Milkovich RN, Hu JCC. Autosomal dominant amelogenesis imperfecta associated with ENAM frameshift mutation p.Asn36Ilefs56. Clin Genet. 2013;83:195–7.

72. Stephanopoulos G, Garefalaki M-E, Lyroudia K. Genes and related proteins involved in amelogenesis imperfecta. J Dent Res. 2005;84:1117–26.

73. Tsuchiya M, Sharma R, Tye CE, Sugiyama T, Bartlett JD. Transforming growth factor-beta1 expression is up-regulated in maturation-stage enamel organ and may induce ameloblast apoptosis. Eur J Oral Sci. 2009;117:105–12.

74. Venezie RD, Vadiakas G, Christensen JR, Wright JT. Enamel pretreatment with sodium hypochlorite to enhance bonding in hypocalcified amelogenesis imperfecta: case report and SEM analysis. Pediatr Dent. 1994;16:433–6.

75. Vitkov L, Hannig M, Krautgartner WD. Restorative therapy of primary teeth severely affected by amelogenesis imperfecta. Quintessence Int. 2006;37:219–24.

76. Weerheijm KL, Groen HJ, Beentjes VE, Poorterman JH. Prevalence of cheese molars in eleven-year-old Dutch children. ASDC J Dent Child. 2001;68:259–62, 229.

77. Weerheijm KL, Jalevik B, Alaluusua S. Molar-incisor hypomineralisation. Caries Res. 2001;35:390–1.

78. William V, Messer LB, Burrow MF. Molar incisor hypomineralization: review and recommendations for clinical management. Pediatr Dent. 2006;28:224–32.

79. Williams WP, Becker LH. Amelogenesis imperfecta: functional and esthetic restoration of a severely compromised dentition. Quintessence Int. 2000;31:397–403.

80. Winter GB. Amelogenesis imperfecta with enamel opacities and taurodontism: an alternative diagnosis for 'idiopathic dental fluorosis'. Br Dent J. 1996;181:167–72.

81. Witkop C. Amelogenesis imperfecta, dentinogenesis imperfecta and dentin dysplasia revisited: problems in classification. J Oral Pathol. 1988;17:547–53.

82. Witkop CJ. Partial expression of sex-linked recessive amelogenesis imperfecta in females compatible with the Lyon hypothesis. Oral Surg Oral Med Oral Pathol. 1967;23:174.

83. Wright J, Hart P, Aldred M, Seow K, Crawford P, Hong S, Gibson C, Hart T. Relationship of phenotype and genotype in X-linked amelogenesis imperfecta. Connect Tissue Res. 2003;44:72–8.

84. Wright J, Waite P, Mueninghoff L, Sarver D. The multidisciplinary approach managing enamel defects. J Am Dent Assoc. 1991;122:62–5.

85. Wright JT. The molecular etiologies and associated phenotypes of amelogenesis imperfecta. Am J Med Genet. 2006;140A:2547–55.

86. Wright JT, Daly B, Simmons D, Hong S, Hart SP, Hart TC, Atsawasuwan P, Yamauchi M. Human enamel phenotype associated with amelogenesis imperfecta and a kallikrein-4 (g.2142G>A) proteinase mutation. Eur J Oral Sci. 2006;114 Suppl 1:13–7; discussion 39–41, 379.

87. Wright JT, Fine J-D, Johnson LB. Developmental defects of enamel in humans with hereditary epidermolysis bullosa. Arch Oral Biol. 1993;38:945–55.

88. Wright JT, Frazier-Bowers S, Simmons D, Alexander K, Crawford P, Han ST, Hart PS, Hart TC. Phenotypic variation in FAM83H-associated amelogenesis imperfecta. J Dent Res. 2009;88:356–60.

89. Wright JT, Hart TC, Hart PS, Simmons D, Suggs C, Daley B, Simmer J, Hu J, Bartlett JD, Li Y, Yuan ZA, Seow WK, Gibson CW. Human and mouse enamel phenotypes resulting from mutation or altered expression of AMEL, ENAM, MMP20 and KLK4. Cells Tissues Organs. 2009;189:224–9.

90. Wright JT, Kula K, Hall K, Simmons JH, Hart TC. Analysis of the tricho-dento-osseous syndrome genotype and phenotype. Am J Med Genet. 1997;72:197–204.

91. Wright JT, Torain M, Long K, Seow K, Crawford P, Aldred MJ, Hart PS, Hart TC. Amelogenesis imperfecta: genotype-phenotype studies in 71 families. Cells Tissues Organs. 2011;194:279–83.

92. Yengopal V, Mickenautsch S. Caries preventive effect of casein phosphopeptide-amorphous calcium phosphate (CPP-ACP): a meta-analysis. Acta Odontol Scand. 2009;67:321–32.

93. Yip HK, Smales RJ. Oral rehabilitation of young adults with amelogenesis imperfecta. Int J Prosthodont. 2003;16:345–9.

Defects of Dentin Development

7

Hani Nazzal and Monty S. Duggal

Abstract

The management of children with defects of dentin can be challenging from both diagnostic and treatment perspectives. Obtaining the correct diagnosis is based on careful evaluation of the family history, clinical manifestations and radiographic appearance. Therefore, this chapter aims at describing the various types of conditions leading to defects in dentin with emphasis on the importance of establishing a holistic treatment plan that encompasses a stepwise approach to help achieve the short-, medium- and long-term treatment goals of a functional and aesthetic dentition.

Introduction

Dentin is a calcified tooth tissue which consists of about 70 % mineral (hydroxyapatite), 20 % organic matrix and 10 % water (mature dentin) [1]. It serves as a protective covering for the pulp while supporting enamel and cementum.

The formation of dentin, a process known as dentinogenesis, is carried out by specialised ectomesenchymally derived cells known as odontoblasts. These columnar cells line the pulpal surface of the dentin with the cell processes extending partly or all the way through dentin. The odontoblasts are associated with the formation and maintenance of dentin and communication with pulp afferent nerves. The odontoblasts provide the tooth with a biological line of defence against environmental injury and the ability to lay down reparative or tertiary dentin in response to insults such as dental caries or tooth fracture.

Defects of dentin can be of genetic origin or caused by environmental effects. The clinical characteristics of these conditions (phenotype) are diverse, and the clinician is challenged by correctly diagnosing the diverse conditions that affect dentin and selecting appropriate treatment approaches. Abnormalities of dentin formation are generally divided into the following:

A. Nonsyndromic defects of dentin, inherited conditions, e.g. dentinogenesis imperfecta and dentinal dysplasia
B. Syndromes with dentin defects
  (a) Osteogenesis imperfecta (OI) with dentinogenesis imperfecta
  (b) Ehlers-Danlos syndrome

H. Nazzal (✉) • M.S. Duggal
Department of Pediatric Dentistry,
Leeds University, Leeds, UK
e-mail: h.abudiak@leeds.ac.uk

J.T. Wright (ed.), *Craniofacial and Dental Developmental Defects: Diagnosis and Management*,
DOI 10.1007/978-3-319-13057-6_7, © Springer International Publishing Switzerland 2015

(c) Goldblatt syndrome
(d) Schimke immuno-osseous dysplasia
(e) Hypophosphataemic rickets, X-linked dominant vitamin D-resistant rickets

Nonsyndromic Dentin Defects: Dentinogenesis Imperfecta and Dentin Dysplasia

Definition

Dentinogenesis imperfecta (DGI) and dentin dysplasia (DD) are inherited conditions in which abnormal dentin structure and composition affect either the primary or both the primary and secondary dentitions. With the exception of DD type I, these conditions are inherited as autosomal dominant traits. De novo mutations in the *DSPP* gene that causes these conditions have been reported but occur very rarely, so in most instances there will be a positive family history. New mutations do occur frequently in the genes that code for type I collagen, so clinicians should be highly suspicious that an individual with an apparent sporadic case of DGI also has OI.

Epidemiology

The incidence of nonsyndromic DGI is reported to be 1 in 6,000 to 1 in 8,000, while that of DD type I is 1 in 100,000 [2].

Classification

The most familiar classification system of DGI and DD is that of Shields 1973 [3] where DGI is divided into three types (DGI-I, GDI-II and DGI-III) and DD into two types (DD-I, DD-II). This classification is widely used, but does not always encompass the range of clinical and radiographic features that can be seen within these groups of defects. This classification system does not take into account the molecular basis of these conditions, and it is now known that DGI types II and III as well as DD type II are all caused by mutations in the *DSPP* gene. As will be discussed, there are

differences in the OMIM and Shields classifications for DGI adding further confusion to the nomenclature for hereditary dentin disorders. The clinical and radiographic features of patients from the Brandywine isolate (DGI-III) showed bulbous crowns with cervical constriction similar to DGI-II [4]; however, they also showed enlarged pulp chambers that became completely obliterated with time. Another case of DGI-III was shown to have odontodysplastic features [5]. DGI-III thus represents a slight phenotypic variant of DGI-II and is managed clinically in a similar manner.

While DD-II, DGI-II and DGI-III show some variability in their clinical phenotype, they are allelic, and different individuals from the same kindred had been found to have different clinical features [6] further suggesting these conditions are variants of the same condition [6].

The most current Online Mendelian Inheritance in Man (OMIM) database classification excludes DGI with osteogenesis imperfecta as one of the types of DGI, and therefore, Shields' DGI-II is now DGI-I (MIM 125490), Shields' DGI-III is now DGI-II (MIM 125500), and Shields' DD-I and DD-II remained the same (MIM 125400 and MIM 125420, respectively).

Despite this change in classification of DGI and DD, the Shields' classification remains the most widely known classification and therefore will be used in this chapter.

Clinical Presentation [2, 3, 7]

Dentinogenesis Imperfecta (Shields Type I – OMIM 166200, 166210)
This DGI type is associated with various forms of the syndrome osteogenesis imperfecta (OI – brittle bone disease). This is usually a result of mutations in one of the two collagen type 1 genes (*COL1A1* and *COL1A2*) although OI is caused by mutations in a variety of genes associated with collagen and fibrillogenesis.

Clinical presentation
The clinical presentation of DGI type I is highly variable, and only about 30 % of individuals with OI will have a DGI phenotype. The primary and permanent teeth are amber and translucent with

the permanent teeth tending to be less affected compared with the primary dentition. The structural defect of the dentin and its decreased level of mineralisation frequently lead to enamel fracturing, which is then followed by significant attrition of the underlying soft dentin. It has often been claimed that this is associated with a smooth enamel dentin junction; however, some studies demonstrated that this was not the case, and enamel loss most likely occurs secondary to the abnormal physical properties of the abnormal dentin.

Radiographical presentation
The teeth can have short, narrow roots with pulpal obliteration occurring either before or just after eruption. This is not always the case as some teeth show total pulpal obliteration, while others appear normal. In rare cases the pulp chambers may be enlarged and subsequently undergo pulp canal obliteration.

Dentinogenesis Imperfecta Type II (Shields Type II – OMIM # 125490) (Fig. 7.1)
This is the isolated nonsyndromic type of DGI and is caused by mutations in the *DSPP* gene. The *DSPP* gene codes for the most abundant of the non-collagenous proteins in dentin.

Clinical presentation
The dental features of this type are similar to those of DGI-I, but penetrance is virtually complete (normal teeth are never found). There might be some variation in the severity of the condition between different members of the same family and individual teeth in the same patient. In addition, the crowns are typically bulbous with marked cervical constriction. The teeth tend to be clinically smaller than unaffected teeth.

Radiographical presentation
Similar to DGI-I.

Dentinogenesis Imperfecta (Shields Type III)
This is also known as the Brandywine isolate type as it was first described in a triracial population from Maryland and Washington DC.

Clinical presentation
This type has variable expressivity with clinical features sometimes resembling those of DGI-I and type II.

Radiographical presentation
The primary teeth appear hollow radiographically due to the lack of dentin formation and very large pulp chambers. As a result of the large pulp chambers, enamel fracturing and rapid dentin wear, these teeth develop multiple pulp exposures and are prone to abscess formation.

Dentin Dysplasia (Shields Type I – OMIM)

Clinical presentation
The dental crowns in DD-I appear generally normal in shape, form and colour. However, the dentin has a pathognomic cascading waterfall histological appearance in thin sections, and the root form is abnormal to varying degrees. The teeth often are displaced or malaligned and have increased mobility. These teeth have an increased risk for developing periapical abscesses in the absence of dental caries or other aetiological factors.

Radiographical presentation
The roots can be sharp with conical, apical constrictions or have extremely short blunt roots. Pre-eruptive pulpal obliteration occurs in both the primary and permanent teeth. Pulpal obliteration is usually complete in the primary teeth; however, it is often only partial in the permanent dentition (crescent-shaped pulpal remnant parallel to the cementoenamel junction). Numerous periapical radiolucencies are often seen in non-carious teeth (Fig. 7.2).

Dentin Dysplasia (Shields Type II – OMIM 125420)

Clinical presentation
The features seen in the deciduous dentition resemble those observed in DGI-II; however, the permanent dentition is either unaffected or shows mild radiographic abnormalities and can have slight colour changes.

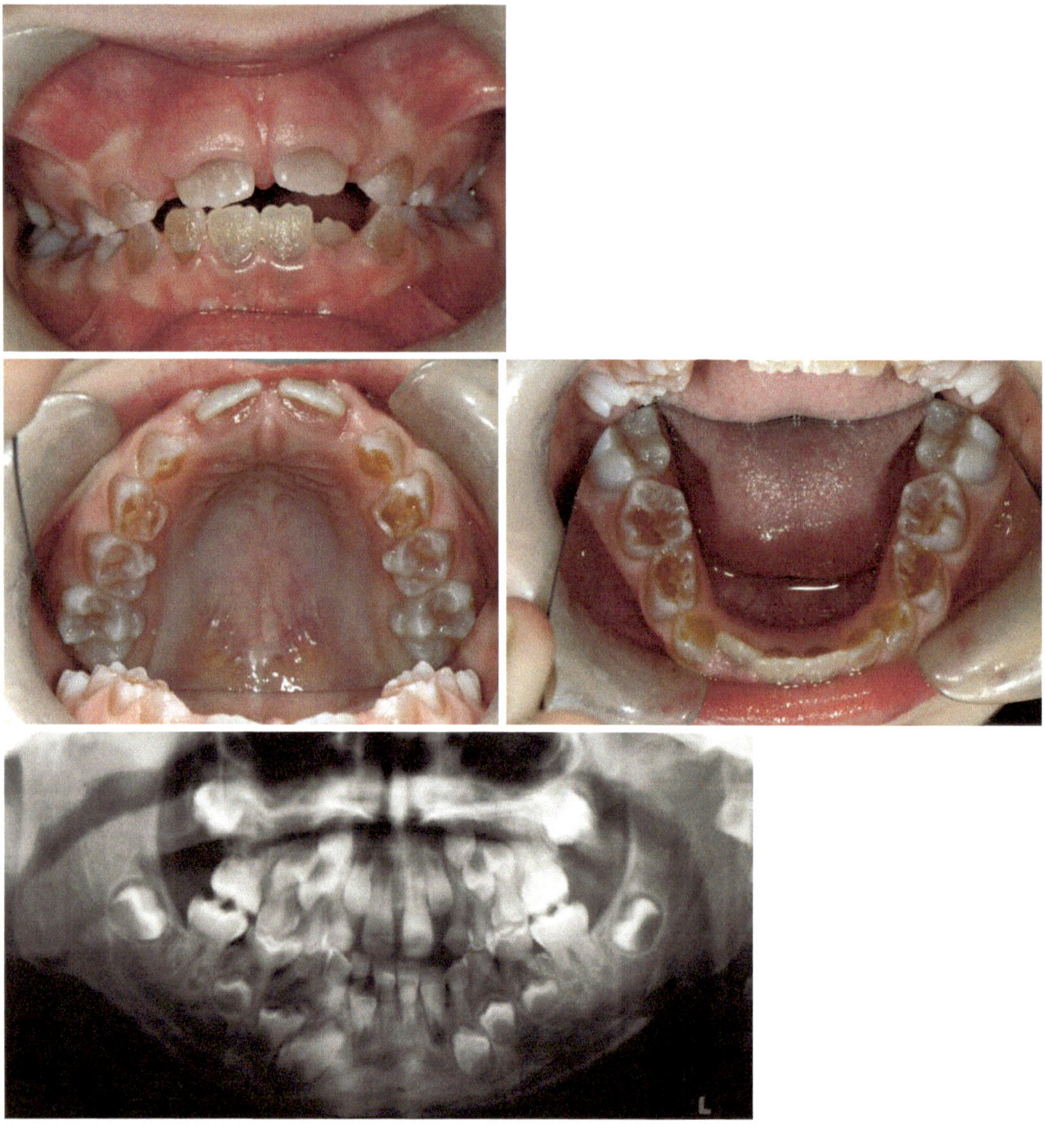

Fig. 7.1 Photographs and an OPG of a patient with type II dentinogenesis imperfecta showing amber primary and permanent teeth with tooth surface loss (enamel fracture and attrition of underlying dentin). The OPT shows short, narrow roots with pulpal obliteration of the primary teeth and the first permanent molars

Fig. 7.2 This individual with DD type I has complete obliteration of all the pulp chambers that is seen to be occurring even in the unerupted third molars. The roots are short, and the mandibular right first permanent molar has developed periapical pathology

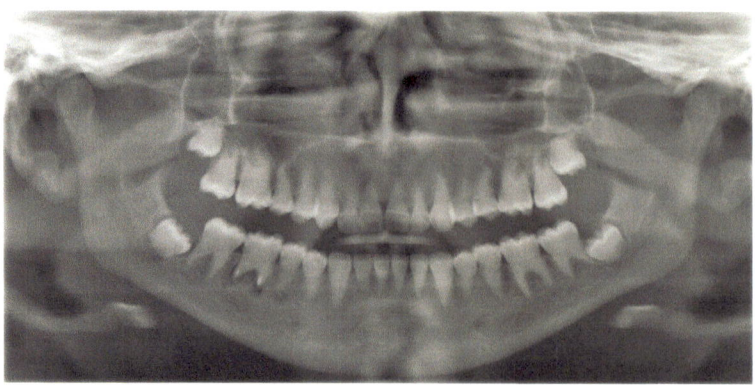

Radiographical presentation
Thistle-tube deformity of the pulp chamber of the permanent teeth and frequent pulp stones.

Molecular Aetiology

The organic component of dentin is composed predominantly of type I collagen (85 %) and non-collagenous protein mainly dentin phosphoprotein (50 %). Numerous genes are involved in regulating the production of the complex dentinal extracellular matrix which eventually mineralises in a highly controlled way.

Type I collagen is the product of *COL1A1* and *COL1A2* genes, while dentin phosphoprotein and dentin sialoprotein (*DSPP*) are products of the *DSPP* gene. There are known to be hundreds of different mutations in *COL1A1* and *COL1A2* genes that are associated with osteogenesis imperfecta; however, only some of the collagen mutations result in dentinogenesis imperfecta. Mutations in either type 1 collagen genes or the *DSPP* gene can alter the essential interactions between these proteins resulting in abnormal mineralisation and a DI dental phenotype.

Syndromic Dentin Defects

Osteogenesis Imperfecta

This condition is usually a result of mutations in one of the two collagen type 1 genes (*COL1A1* and *COL1A2*). This condition is transmitted as an autosomal dominant or autosomal recessive trait, and there are multiple types of OI. The most common classification [8] lists four subtypes, but there are now over ten listed on OMIM. The severity varies markedly between different individuals and families. These OI conditions are characterised by bone fragility, blue sclera, deafness mainly at third decade of life and lax ligaments (hypermobility of joints). In severe cases, there can be marked bony deformities, including scoliosis, compression fractions of the vertebrae and ribs, short stature, frontal bossing and other manifestations. Dentinogenesis imperfecta can be a manifestation of osteogenesis imperfecta.

Many individuals with severe forms of OI will be treated with intravenous bisphosphonate treatments to try and improve bone density and decrease the risk of fractures. While IV bisphosphonate treatment has been associated with bone necrosis following dental extractions, there have not been cases of this problem reported in OI patients.

Ehlers-Danlos Syndrome (EDS)

Ehlers-Danlos syndrome is the most common of the heritable connective tissue disorders. It consists of nine major variants with inheritance patterns of either autosomal dominant or recessive, depending on the type. The clinical manifestations in the different EDS conditions result from defects in the synthesis, secretion or polymerisation of collagen. The main features of EDS include tissue fragility, skin extensibility and joint hypermobility.

Defective dentinogenesis affecting the mandibular incisors was reported in some EDS type I where aplasia or hypoplasia of root development, bulbous enlargement of the roots and pulp stones were reported [9]. Others reported dental features such as dysplastic dentin and obliterated pulp chambers [10].

EDS type VIII (OMIM # 130080) is associated with severe early-onset periodontitis that is managed with aggressive local debridement and antibiotic therapy.

Goldblatt Syndrome (OMIM # 184260)

Goldblatt syndrome, also known as spondylometaphyseal dysplasia, is characterised by joint laxity, mesomelic limb shortening and DGI. The deciduous teeth display typical features of DGI, but the permanent teeth appear normal [11].

Schimke Immuno-Osseous Dysplasia (OMIM # 242900)

Schimke immuno-osseous dysplasia is an autosomal recessive disorder caused by mutations in the

SMARCAL1 gene. It is characterised by a combination of spondyloepiphyseal dysplasia, progressive renal disease and lymphopenia with defective cellular immunity [11]. Patients with this condition were also reported to have dental features of DGI, such as a grey-yellowish discoloration of the dentin, bulbous crowns with a marked cervical constriction and small or obliterated pulp chambers [11].

Hypophosphataemic Rickets, X-Linked Dominant Vitamin D-Resistant Rickets (OMIM # 307800)

X-linked dominant hypophosphataemic rickets is one of the types of rickets where patients have bone deformities, short stature and hypophosphataemia. Hypophosphataemia is the result of mutations in the phosphate-regulating gene on the X chromosome that results in renal wasting of phosphorus at the proximal tubule level. These patients, therefore, are characterised by low renal phosphate reabsorption, normal serum calcium level with hypocalciuria, normal or low serum level of vitamin D (1,25(OH)2D3, or calcitriol), normal serum level of PTH and increased activity of serum alkaline phosphatases [7, 12].

Dentally, the dentine is the most markedly affected tissue in these patients. They present clinically with dental abscesses in the absence of caries, radiographically with larger pulp chambers and elongated pulp horns and histopathologically with interglobular dentine. Dental attrition can lead to exposure of the large pulp horns causing loss of vitality and abscesses [7, 13].

Management of Defects in Dentin Formation

The management of individuals with defects of dentin can be challenging from both diagnostic and treatment perspectives. Obtaining the diagnosis is based on careful evaluation of the family history, clinical manifestations and radiographic appearance. A genetics consultation should be considered

for dentin defects that appear to be hereditary. Management often requires immediate-, short- and long-term planning. The long-term management of these patients usually requires an interdisciplinary approach starting in the primary/early mixed dentition.

Patients with dentinal defects of primary teeth often present at a young age with parents wanting immediate treatment to improve the child's appearance or because the teeth are beginning to develop abscesses. However, it is important to make a treatment plan which will encompass a stepwise approach that includes a vision to help achieve the short-, medium- and long-term treatment goals of a functional and aesthetic dentition. Children with dentinal defects often require several interventions throughout their primary, mixed and possibly permanent dentition stages. Should general anaesthesia (GA) be required to provide extensive restorative/surgical treatments, it is crucial to plan and provide the necessary management in a timely manner so that the least number of GAs are required throughout the child's life.

The goals of oral health management, especially at the primary dentition stage, include the following:

1. Obtaining a diagnosis of the condition if it is unknown
2. Prevention and maintenance of good oral hygiene
3. Desensitisation and pain management of affected teeth (if required)
4. Restorative management (aesthetic management and stabilisation of affected teeth)
5. Behaviour management to help children manage the dental care they need

General Management

Need for Early Detection

Early detection of tooth structural defects such as DGI, DD and amelogenesis imperfecta is of great importance for multiple reasons. These conditions can be associated with other more serious conditions such as osteogenesis imperfecta and vitamin D deficiency which would allow early detection of these conditions. Additionally, some of these conditions are associated with tooth surface, possible pulp exposure or periapical infections, therefore; early detection would allow close monitoring of these cases and early intervention and prevention where needed.

Care should be taken not to confuse these cases with other conditions with similar clinical presentation such as [2]:

1. Amelogenesis imperfecta where enamel defects causes enamel loss and exposure of underlying dentin (Fig. 7.3)
2. Intrinsic discolouration resembling amber/translucent colour:
   (a) Red-brown discolouration due to haemolytic anaemia such as congenital erythropoietic porphyria and rhesus incompatibility
   (b) Yellow or grey to brown discolouration such as tetracycline stain

(c) Green discolouration: Hyperbilirubinaemia such as in cases of congenital biliary atresia (Fig. 7.4), acute liver failure and biliary hypoplasia
3. Mobility leading to early tooth loss resembling teeth lost in DGI-III and DD-I due to periapical abscesses and short roots such as:
   (a) Hypophosphatasia
   (b) Immunological deficiencies, e.g. severe congenital neutropenia, cyclic neutropaenia, Chediak-Higashi syndrome, neutropaenias, histiocytosis X, Papillon-Lefevre syndrome and leucocyte adhesion deficiency syndrome

Assessment of Medical History

A medical history should aim to establish if the dental condition is a 'syndromic' form of DGI as this is a variable feature of a number of heritable conditions as discussed previously. For instance,

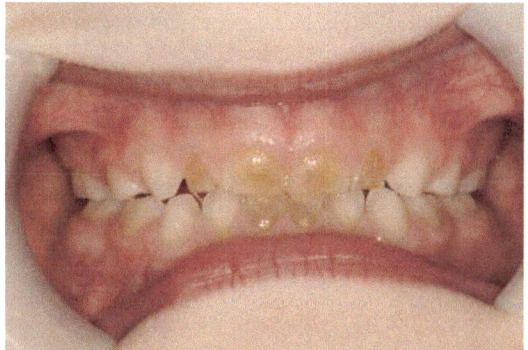
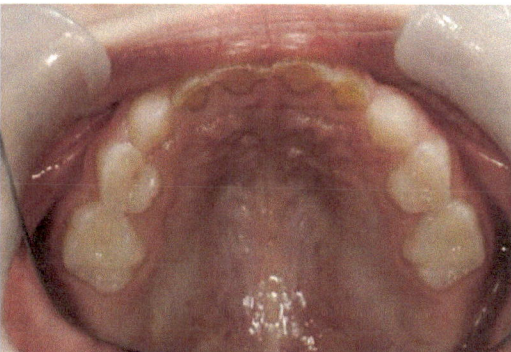
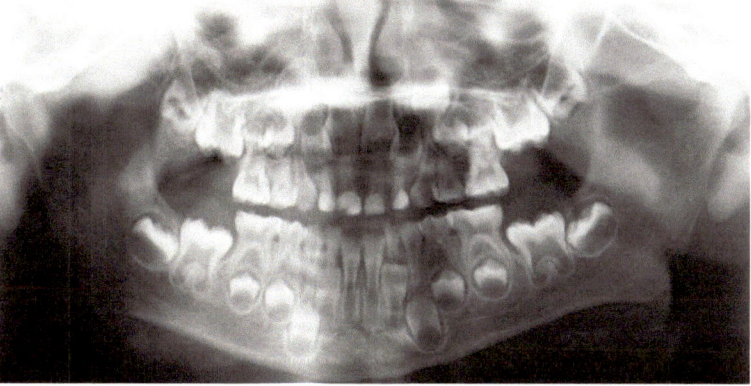

Fig. 7.3 Photograph of a patient with hypomineralised amelogenesis imperfecta with amber upper and lower anterior primary teeth. OPT showed no difference in radiodensity of enamel and dentin on all anterior teeth and all Ds in addition to reduced radiopacity of the enamel on posterior teeth suggestive of amelogenesis imperfecta

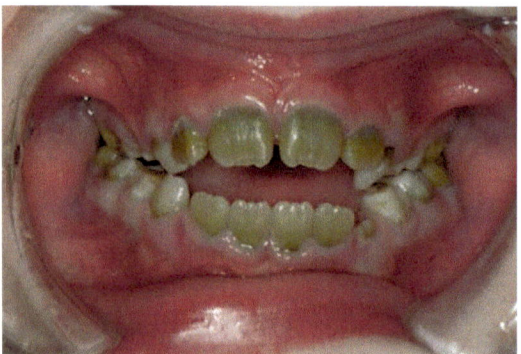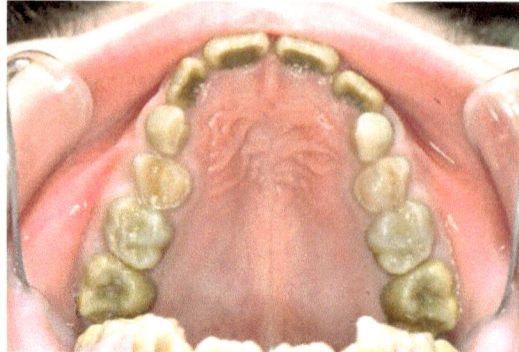

Fig. 7.4 Photographs of a patient with biliary atresia showing green discolouration of primary and permanent teeth due to hyperbilirubinaemia

patients with DGI should be checked for history of bone fractures with minimal trauma, joint hyperextensibility, short stature, hearing loss and scleral hue in order to help exclude osteogenesis imperfecta. This is especially important in what appear to be sporadic cases of DGI that have no family history.

This is important as the overall dental management of these patients should take into account other associated medical conditions such as OI, hypophosphataemic rickets, EDS, etc. For instance, patients with EDS can have different complications depending on the type of EDS such as fragile skin tissues, structural heart defects, poor wound healing, hypermobility of the joints and fragile blood vessels. It is therefore important to liaise carefully with the patient's physician in order to determine the exact type and the associated risks prior to arranging any dental treatments.

Patients with OI and hypophosphataemic rickets are susceptible to bone fractures, and therefore, physical restraint is contraindicated in these patients. In addition, manual handling of these patients under GA should be performed with extreme care.

Furthermore, over the last decade bisphosphonates are being increasingly used in children and adolescents especially for the management of OI. Although bisphosphonates are well tolerated, concerns exist regarding bisphosphonate-related osteonecrosis of the jaw or BRONJ. BRONJ has been defined as 'a condition of exposed bone in the mandible or maxilla that persists for more than 8 weeks in a patient who has taken or currently is taking a bisphosphonate and who has no history of radiation therapy to the jaw' [14]. Trauma, either surgical or from a prosthesis in patients taking bisphosphonates, is the key factor causing the condition. Oral bisphosphonates are seldom associated with BRONJ, and it is the intravenous use that remains a concern for this condition.

Although there have been no cases of BRONJ reported in children or adolescents, in addition to reports showing no development of BRONJ in children receiving bisphosphonates following surgical interventions [14], it is imperative that clinicians should liaise with their medical colleagues in the management of these patients. Although there are no available evidence-based guidelines for the management of children and adolescents, the following should be considered in the management of these patients [14].

Prior to using bisphosphonates children should receive the following:

1. Comprehensive clinical and radiographic dental assessment aimed at the elimination of any foci of oral infection.
2. Rigorous preventive programme to prevent further caries and obviate the need for any surgical intervention.
3. No elective surgical procedures. Such procedures should be deferred for as long as practically possible after completion of bisphosphonate treatment.

During a course of bisphosphonates:

1. Delay any surgical intervention as long as possible from the last bisphosphonate infusion.
2. Use 0.12 % chlorhexidine gluconate mouth rinse and local antiseptic measures before and after surgery.
3. Surgical intervention should be as conservative as possible, and a healing period of 3 weeks should be allowed prior to the next bisphosphonate infusion.
4. Extraction sockets or surgical wounds should be sutured wherever possible.
5. Prophylactic antibiotics should only be considered for those children deemed to be at highest risk for BRONJ, such as immune-compromised children.
6. Close monitoring of the surgical site for up to 12 months postoperatively.

Genetic Counselling

A family history should establish which other members are affected and allow a pedigree to be completed. Dentinogenesis imperfecta and dentinal dysplasia are inherited in an autosomal dominant fashion; therefore, there is a 50 % chance the offspring of an affected individual will be affected. There can also be male to male transmission of the condition which does not occur in X-linked conditions like X-linked vitamin D-resistant rickets (OMIM # 307800). Achieving a diagnosis is predicated on sound clinical findings, and then genetic counselling can be useful where there is doubt of the type of dentinal defect and where confirmation of association with other syndromes is suspected.

Prevention

Although caries is typically not a major issue in these patients (the teeth often wear down faster than they can become carious), prevention is paramount to prevent caries from adding to existing problems. Enamel loss especially in DGI-I and II can lead to dentin exposure. This can lead to tooth sensitivity and increases the patients' caries risk. Therefore, treatment planning should firstly focus on prevention including effective oral hygiene instruction using soft brushes, optimising fluoride

exposure both at home and with regular professional application, diet advice and fissure sealant application or temporary restorations where appropriate. A guide is given in the UK Department of Health and British Association for the Study of Community Dentistry Toolkit [15]. Comprehensive dietary analysis and advice are essential from both caries and tooth surface loss perspectives. This will involve identifying fermentable carbohydrates and acidic foods and beverages in the diet and advising on their reduction to minimise damage.

Reducing Sensitivity

Patients with exposed dentin can develop sensitivity associated with cold and hot food and drinks. This sensitivity can make restorative interventions, especially with adhesive materials even more challenging. Some of the suggested methods for desensitisation include the use of topical fluoride preparations, in particular fluoride varnishes, such as Duraphat® 22,600 ppm F (Colgate Oral Care) or 3 M Espe fluoride varnish with tricalcium phosphate.

More recently a combination of casein phosphopeptide and amorphous calcium phosphate (CPP-ACP – GC Tooth Mousse/MI Paste) with and without fluoride has also been advocated to help decrease sensitivity. CPP-ACP helps create, stabilise and deposit a super saturated solution of calcium and phosphate at the enamel surface. Therefore, it has been suggested that home application of a CPP-ACP containing cream especially when combined with fluoride use will help remineralise and desensitise by acting as a source of bioavailable calcium and phosphate. Other topical fluorides may also be useful; amongst these are stannous fluoride gels, such as Gel-Kam® 1,000 ppm F (Colgate Oral Care) or OMNI Gel 0.4 %/1,000 ppmF (3 M). There has also been a suggestion that desensitising toothpastes may help with some of these teeth. For example, toothpastes containing NovaMin have been clinically shown to help reduce dental sensitivity associated with exposed dentin. However, none of the available products are always effective, and clinicians should consider using products in combination or trying different products in an attempt to alleviate patients' symptoms. In severe cases of dental sensitivity due to exposed dentin, full coverage crowns will often be the treatment of choice.

Pain and Anxiety Management

Pain management in children is an integral part of good paediatric dentistry. Both the technique and choice of local analgesia are important for the provision of high quality, effective restorations in children, particularly if they are to last for the lifetime of the primary teeth (up to 8 years).

Behaviour Management

Children with dentinal defects often present for treatment at a young age and with the expected age-appropriate levels of anxiety. This is especially true in cases where the defect is associated with sensitivity or where previous treatment has been attempted without appropriate pain control or behaviour management. If such defects are suspected, especially when associated with sensitivity, it is important not to air dry these teeth during examination but to dry them gently with cotton pellet.

Managing young children requires empathy and knowledge of behaviour management techniques for children. Many paediatric dentistry textbooks cover useful techniques for helping children cope with restorative care. In the centre of all the techniques is 'tell, show and do' which will allow most children to be able to cooperate for restorative care when it is presented in age-appropriate language and demonstration. This of course takes a little extra time but is time well spent in preparing a child for more complex care as they grow older.

Local Analgesia

For children who have been sensitised to previous invasive dental treatment, in particular local analgesia, the use of computer-controlled anaesthesia (such as the WAND and the WAND STA – Controlled Dental Anaesthesia, Dental Practice Systems, Welwyn, Herts, UK) can be an excellent way to administer local analgesia. The WAND provides several advantages over conventional syringes including the fact that it does

not look like a conventional syringe; the fine bevel of the needle and the slow speed with which the local analgesic solution can be administered make it a simple way to deliver painless local analgesia. Some researchers found the WAND to significantly reduce disruptive behaviours during the initial 15 s of the injection [16]; however, others showed no difference in the pain or anxiety experienced by the children between the WAND and the traditional local analgesic techniques [17].

The use of 4 % articaine should be considered in managing older children especially where there is a history of failed local analgesia. For children over 4 years of age who are extremely wary of local analgesia, infiltration with 4 % articaine in the lower arch as opposed to an inferior dental block may provide adequate analgesia for restorations to be placed [18]. It is also important to make use of topical anaesthesia. The pre-emptive use of systemic analgesics (in accordance with local guidelines) can also be an effective way of helping children cope with care successfully.

Sedation

In extremely apprehensive children who are otherwise cooperative, the use of inhalation sedation should be considered. This form of sedation has the particular benefit of having an analgesic effect which lessens the child's response to painful stimuli. Hence for children whose apprehension is due to sensitive teeth that have been previously treated without effective local analgesia, inhalation sedation with nitrous oxide and oxygen provides a safe, effective and a noninvasive method for managing the child's anxiety [19]. Other forms of sedation can be utilised according to local guidelines and clinicians' usual practice.

General Anaesthesia

Children with severe dentinal defects often present before they are old enough to cope with restorative dentistry; therefore, the use of general anaesthesia is effective and valid for this group. Clinicians treating children with severe dentinal defects especially those with sensitive teeth or those with bad dental experience should consider the early use of general anaesthesia to allow effective successful stabilisation of the primary teeth. Previous studies of treatment under general anaesthesia have shown good outcomes with decrease in the numbers of repeat restorations [20].

Management of Primary Teeth with Dentinal Defects

The aims of management of primary dentition in patients with dentinal defects include maintaining dental health, function and vertical dimension, preserving tooth vitality, improving aesthetic appearance in order to prevent psychological problems and establishing rapport with the patient and the patient's family early in the treatment [21].

The decision to restore primary teeth with dentinal defects depends on several factors:

1. Type of dentinal defect. DGI usually affects both primary and permanent teeth; however, the effect is usually less severe in permanent teeth evident by tooth surface loss [22]. DGI-III is associated with early pulp exposures leading to loss of vitality; therefore, early full coverage might be advisable. DD-I is associated with short rooted primary teeth leading to tooth mobility, and there is no specific treatment for this condition.
2. Extent and severity of the defects. Some cases might involve significant tooth surface loss, which will suggest that more radical restorative/extraction options can be considered.
3. Associated symptoms. In cases of severe sensitivity, full coverage should be considered.
4. Aesthetics with possible psychological effects on the child. The psychological impact of these conditions in children should never be underestimated. Aesthetic management should be offered as soon as the child and the parents wish to have this carried out.
5. Patient cooperation and the method of treatment. In children who cannot cope with treatment under local analgesia, alternative strategies such as sedation or general anaesthesia should be considered.

Interim Restorations

In some cases it may be appropriate to place interim therapeutic restorations to immediately alleviate pain and sensitivity and to prevent further tooth wear while awaiting more definitive restorative treatment. The provision of these interim restorations also allows the clinician to establish a rapport with the child and assist in behaviour management. Materials such as resin-modified glass ionomer can be useful as these materials incorporate appropriate bonding for both enamel and any exposed dentin. Some of the materials also incorporate a colour that allows good visualisation of the extent of the restoration on the tooth surface, e.g. Fuji VII/Triage (GC Corporation). The release of fluoride from these materials, although not proven to be a major factor, may also help to reduce sensitivity by encouraging further mineralisation of the surrounding enamel.

Compomer materials (polyacid-modified composite) might also be considered and can be placed using self-etching primers. These materials have the advantage of being more wear resistant than glass ionomer cement-based materials and have dual-bonding technology, which may seal both enamel and dentin effectively especially when further sealed with adhesive resin or fissure sealant following placement.

Longer-Term Restorations
Composite Resin Restorations

Composite veneers placed at the chairside should be considered for the restoration of primary anterior teeth [21].

In posterior teeth, composite resin should be considered in cases where enamel loss:
- Does not involve cusp tips.
- There is no significant tooth wear or sensitivity.
- Margins of the defects are supragingival.

Preformed Crowns

Full coverage with either stainless steel or other aesthetic preformed crowns should be considered in cases where:
- The defect involves multiple surfaces.
- There is significant tooth wear and sensitivity.
- There is involvement of the cusp tips in posterior teeth.

- Severe enamel chipping and exposed dentin.
- Treatment has to be carried out under general anaesthesia, and the child is unlikely to manage restorative care in the immediate future.

While preformed metal crowns (stainless steel crowns) are a well-recognised option for the treatment of carious primary molars, they also have an important role in the management of patients with dentin defects affecting the primary molars (Fig. 7.5). Placement of stainless steel crowns requires minimal tooth preparation. They are less bulky than the white preformed crowns that may suffer wear and chipping of the veneer.

More recently for very young children, a technique, known as the 'Hall Technique', has been described in which stainless steel crowns are placed with no preparation [23]. While this technique is promoted for children presenting with dental caries, anecdotal reports suggest using this technique to place stainless steel crowns over primary first and second molars

soon after enamel loss is evident is a successful way of managing these teeth. Furthermore adopting this technique means that young children can be treated, without resorting to general anaesthesia, early in the dental chair without local analgesia. Full coverage crowns should be considered in young patients once enamel begins to fracture from the teeth as this will often lead to the rapid attrition and potential loss of the dentition. Long-term studies of the use of stainless steel crowns for carious teeth would suggest that crowns placed over teeth with dentinal defects have advantages over other restorative materials [24]:

1. Perform better where more than two surfaces are affected.
2. Less tooth removal is required.
3. Failure rate is much less than other restorative materials.
4. Moisture control is less critical than when restoring with other materials.

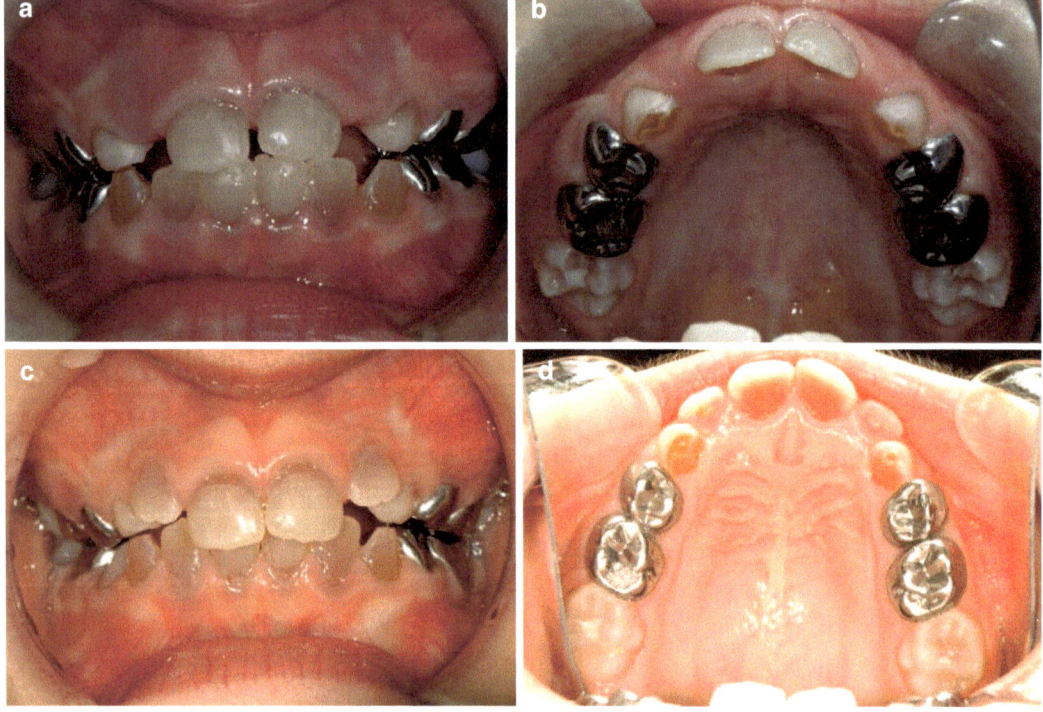

Fig. 7.5 Photographs of a patient with DGI-II (preoperative photos in Fig. 7.1) (**a, b**) following restoration of anterior teeth using composite resin restoration, preformed metal crowns on primary molars and fissure sealants in first permanent molars. (**c, d**) Several months following treatment showing further eruption of anterior teeth and need for further restoration with composite resin

5. Placement is less time consuming than resin restorations.
6. Are more cost-effective as shown by the outcomes over time.
7. Could be used in very young children without the need for a general anaesthesia.

Extraction of Primary Teeth with DDE

In some cases, extractions of severely affected teeth may be required. This should be done with evaluation of the space requirements in the developing dentition. In children where multiple teeth are affected and extractions are required, an interdisciplinary approach involving an orthodontist should be considered to optimise development of the permanent dentition occlusion. Wherever possible, preventive and restorative approaches should be the preferred option as this always gives the child and their family a positive dental health message, where preservation of teeth is considered important.

Management of Permanent Teeth

The principles for the management of the permanent dentition are generally similar to those when restoring the primary teeth. Fortunately in most cases of DGI, the permanent teeth seem to be less susceptible to rapid tooth wear compared with the primary dentition (Fig. 7.6). However, the situation should be monitored closely by regular reviews as once the enamel chips off tooth wear

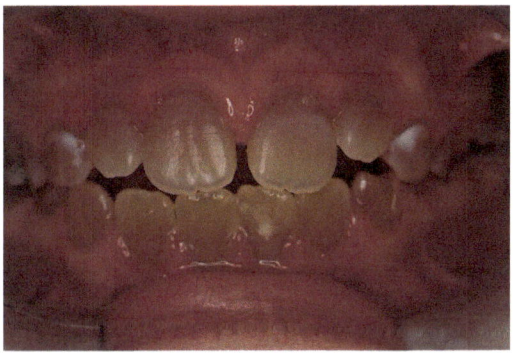

Fig. 7.6 DGI-II showing minimal tooth wear in the permanent teeth. These teeth often do well in the long term but need careful monitoring

can follow rapidly. Intracoronal restorations in permanent teeth that demonstrate enamel fracturing and wear tend not to be as reliable and long-lived as stainless steel crowns. Ultimately aesthetic crowns such as zirconium, porcelain fused to metal or other materials may be indicated.

Management of Permanent Anterior Teeth in Children and Adolescents

In the author's opinion the aesthetic aspirations of the child and family should be carefully weighed against considering the risk-benefit of an invasive approach. Any restoration that might compromise the pulpal integrity of the tooth should never be considered before the age of 16–17. Modern composites allow the provision of acceptable aesthetic restorations in the developing child and the family's aesthetic demands although understandable should be carefully discussed. Inevitably composite restorations have to be replaced several times during the period of growth and development. Also, many children with this condition need constant support to maintain their oral hygiene, especially if the defects are associated with sensitivity. However, composites even if required to be placed often are a better option than laboratory-formed restorations which would need extensive tooth preparation of anterior teeth and therefore should seldom be considered in this age group. If the teeth are markedly discoloured, the use of opaque resins will aid in masking the discoloration. The use of opaque resins is especially helpful in the cervical area where the resin will be thinner. Traditional translucent resins tend to have significant shine-through and will not provide optimal aesthetic results for teeth with dark yellow-brown or blue-grey colouration.

Management of Permanent Posterior Teeth in Children and Adolescents

If full coverage is considered appropriate, the use of permanent molar stainless steel crowns should be considered. Although, this is the least aesthetic option, the longevity and ease of placement make this an ideal way to obtain full coverage (Fig. 7.6).

There are also several options which do not require extensive tooth preparation and in some cases no tooth preparation at all. For premolars lab-formed dentin-bonded crowns, made from composite resin, can sometimes be considered. These require minimal tooth preparation and can be bonded to the tooth with composite resin. These can provide excellent aesthetic results while also providing protection against tooth wear (Fig. 7.7).

For the first and second permanent molars, lab-formed gold onlays with sandblasted bonding surfaces can be used (Fig. 7.8). These also require minimal tooth preparation and can be finished at the contact point proximally. Sandblasted internal surface provides excellent retention when these crowns are cemented with a suitable material such as Panavia $F_{2.0}$ (Kuraray America, Inc, New York, USA)

Summary

Individuals with generalised dentin defects not only require professional technical expertise but also our empathy and understanding of growth and development. Immediate- and short-term restorations aimed at improving aesthetics and protecting teeth against tooth wear should be followed by careful long-term treatment planning, often requiring interdisciplinary approach. Transition from paediatric dentistry to adult restorative care should also be meticulously planned and carried out. By following the basic principles of good restorative care, and growth and development, dentists can make an important contribution to the quality of life of children who are unfortunate enough to manifest these defects.

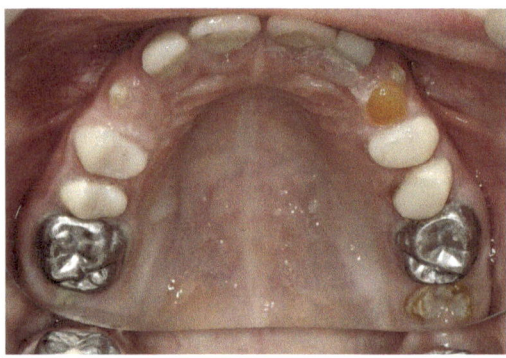

Fig. 7.7 DGI-II showing the use of lab-formed composite crowns for the premolars. Also note the use of stainless steel crowns for the first permanent molars

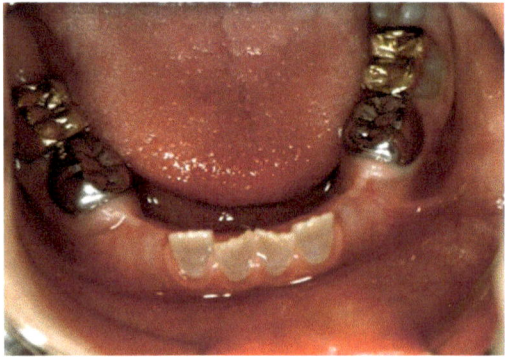

Fig. 7.8 DGI-II showing the use of stainless steel crown for the second primary molars and gold onlays for the first permanent molars

References

1. Nanci A. Dentin-pulp complex. St. Louis: Mosby Elsevier; 2008.
2. Barron MJ, McDonnell ST, Mackie I, Dixon MJ. Hereditary dentin disorders: dentinogenesis imperfecta and dentin dysplasia. Orphanet J Rare Dis. 2008;3:31.
3. Shields ED BD, El-Kafrawy AM. A proposed classification for heritable human dentin defects with a description of a new entity. Arch Oral Biol. 1973;18:543–53.
4. Levin LS, Leaf SH, Jelmini RJ, Rose JJ, Rosenbaum KN. Dentinogenesis imperfecta in the Brandywine isolate (DI type III): clinical, radiologic, and scanning electron microscopic studies of the dentition. Oral Surg Oral Med Oral Pathol. 1983;56:267–74.
5. Clergeau-Guerithault S, Jasmin JR. Dentinogenesis imperfecta type III with enamel and cementum defects. Oral Surg Oral Med Oral Pathol. 1985;59:505–10.
6. Beattie ML, Kim JW, Gong SG, Murdoch-Kinch CA, Simmer JP, Hu JC. Phenotypic variation in dentinogenesis imperfecta/dentin dysplasia linked to 4q21. J Dent Res. 2006;85:329–33.
7. Welbury R, Gillgrass T. Craniofacial growth and development. In: Welbury R, Duggal M, Hosey M,

editors. Paediatric dentistry. 4th ed. Oxford: Oxford University Press; 2012.

8. Sillence DO, Senn A, Danks DM. Genetic heterogeneity in osteogenesis imperfecta. J Med Genet. 1979;16:101–16.

9. Pope FM, Komorowska A, Lee KW, et al. Ehlers Danlos syndrome type I with novel dental features. J Oral Pathol Med. 1992;21:418–21.

10. Barabas GM. The Ehlers-Danlos syndrome. Abnormalities of the enamel, dentin, cementum and the dental pulp: an histological examination of 13 teeth from 6 patients. Br Dent J. 1969;126:509–15.

11. Kim JW, Simmer JP. Hereditary dentin defects. J Dent Res. 2007;86:392–9.

12. Nield LS, Mahajan P, Joshi A, Kamat D. Rickets: not a disease of the past. Am Fam Physician. 2006;74:619–26.

13. Hypophosphatemic Rickets, X-Linked Dominant; XLHR [database on the Internet]. 2014. Available from: http://omim.org/entry/307800?search=RICKE TS&highlight=ricket.

14. Bhatt R, Hibbert S, Munns C. The use of bisphosphonates in children: review of the literature and guidelines for dental management. Aust Dent J. 2014;59:1–11.

15. Department of Health and British Association for the study of Community Dentistry. Delivering Better Oral Health. An evidence-based toolkit for prevention. London: Department of Health; 2009.

16. Gibson R, Allen K, Huftless S, Beiraghi S. The Wand vs traditional injections: a comparison of pain related behaviors. Pediatr Dent. 2000;21:458–62.

17. Tahmassebi J, Nikolaou M, Duggal M. A comparison of pain and anxiety associated with the administration of maxillary local analgesia with Wand and conventional technique. Eur Arch Paediatr Dent. 2009;10:77–82.

18. Leith R, Lynch K, O'Connell A. Articaine use in children: a review. Eur Arch Paediatr Dent. 2012;13:293–6.

19. Paterson S, Tahmassebi J. Paediatric dentistry in the new millenium: 3. Use of inhalation sedation in paediatric dentistry. Dent Update. 2003;30:350–8.

20. Drummond B, Davidson L, Williams S, Moffat S, Ayers K. Outcomes two, three and four years after comprehensive care under general anaesthesia. N Z Dent J. 2004;100:32–7.

21. Sapir S, Shapira J. Dentinogenesis imperfecta: an early treatment strategy. Pediatr Dent. 2001;23:232–7.

22. Rao S, Witkop CJ Jr. Inherited defects in tooth structure. Birth Defects Original Article Series. 1971;7:153–84.

23. Innes NP, Evans DJ, Stirrups DR. The Hall technique; a randomized controlled clinical trial of a novel method of managing carious primary molars in general dental practice: acceptability of the technique and outcomes at 23 months. BMC Oral Health. 2007;7:18.

24. Innes NP, Evans DJ, Stirrups DR. Sealing caries in primary molars: randomized control trial, 5-year results. J Dent Res. 2011;90:1405–10.

Management of Patients with Orofacial Clefts

8

Luiz Pimenta

Abstract

Orofacial clefts (OFCs) are common and treatable birth defects. The etiologies of facial clefts include hereditary, environmental, and multifactorial causes. The role of dentistry in treating individuals with cleft and craniofacial anomalies is to provide comprehensive preventative and therapeutic oral health care. The diversity of surgical and complexity habilitating individuals with facial clefts often necessitates that the dentist work with a team of experts. The use of different services and interventions and their timing are critical to achieve optimal health outcomes in cleft patients. Management of patients from birth to adulthood will be presented and discussed with the main goal to provide the best care and improve the quality of their lives.

Introduction

Orofacial clefts are congenital malformations are characterized by incomplete formation of structures involving the nasal and oral cavities: the lip, alveolus, and hard and soft palate. OFCs vary in size, ranging from a defect of the soft palate or lip only to a complete cleft that extends through the bone (alveolus and hard palate). Since the development and fusion of the lips and the palate occurs at different times, the child could present with a cleft lip only, cleft palate only, or the combination of both, resulting in different variations of OFCs such as (a) cleft lip also known as cheiloschisis, (b) cleft palate or palatoschisis, (c) cleft lip and palate or cheilopalatoschisis, and submucous cleft palate.

Oral cleft is a defect during the development of the frontonasal process where the nose, superior lip, maxilla, and primary palate take origin; another possibility for the occurrence of a cleft is the defect of the fusion of the frontonasal process with the two maxillary processes. These anomalies have their origin at the neural tube.

The pathogenesis of cleft lip and cleft palate is complex; the most widely accepted model is the multifactorial inheritance [1], according to which this pathology is connected to the

L. Pimenta, DDS, MS, PhD (✉)
Clinical Professor, Dental Director – Craniofacial Center – UNC, Department of Dental Ecology, School of Dentistry, University of North Carolina, Chapel Hill, NC, USA
e-mail: Luiz_Pimenta@unc.edu

interaction of genetic and environmental factors [2]. Craniofacial defects such as cleft lip and cleft palate can occur as an isolated condition or may be one component of an inherited disease or syndrome [3]. More than half of patients with OFCs have other associated congenital anomalies [4].

Oral clefts are associated with chromosomal anomalies about 15 % of the time and with monogenic etiologies in about 6 % of cases (about 20 % of cases today are thus known to have genetically testable cause). The number of genes that have been identified with facial clefting syndromes and isolated clefts continues to increase with many listed on OMIM. The search for cleft palate in the OMIM data base results in 683 hits for conditions and genes associated with cleft palate. While many of these conditions do not yet have a known genetic defect, our knowledge of genes associated with clefting has advanced dramatically over the past decade and will continue to do so. Some of the genes identified as causing cleft palate are also associated with missing teeth (e.g., *MSX1* OMIM #142983) and malformed teeth (e.g., *TP63* OMIM #603273).

Orofacial clefts (OFCs) are common and treatable birth defects. Nonsyndromic orofacial cleft (NSOFC) is the most common congenital malformation affecting on average about 1 in 500–750 live newborns annually worldwide [5]. Isolated cleft lip or cleft lip in association with cleft of the palate is the second most common congenital condition in the USA, with an adjusted prevalence of 10.63 per 10,000 live births or 1 in 940 live births [6].

It has been shown that the incidence of cleft lip, with or without cleft palate, varies depending on the ethnicity, and also its prevalence is higher in developing countries [7, 8]. The etiology of cleft lip and/or palate is still largely unknown. The majority of clefts of the lip and palate are believed to have a multifactorial etiology with several genetic and environmental factors interacting to shift the complex process of morphogenesis of the primary and secondary palates toward a threshold of abnormality at which clefting can occur [9].

African Americans have a lower prevalence rate of CL or CLP when compared to Caucasians [6]. Also, a lower prevalence of cleft palate among infants of Hispanic mothers has been reported [10, 11], but not supported by previous studies [12]. Cleft lip with or without cleft palate has a lower prevalence in infants of non-Hispanic Black mothers compared with non-Hispanic and HIspanic White mothers [11–14].

Risk factors that have been identified with cleft palate include maternal behavior (including alcohol and tobacco use) [15, 16], nutrition (e.g., vitamin B6 deficiency), and multiple environmental exposures [17]. Despite the variability of cause, the effect of a cleft palate on naso-oropharyngeal function is similar. The inability to separate the naso-oropharyngeal cavities results in feeding difficulties, speech unintelligibility, and maxillary growth abnormalities [18].

Multi- and Interdisciplinary Team Approach

The role of dentistry in treating individuals with cleft and craniofacial anomalies is to provide comprehensive preventative and therapeutic oral health care.

Treatment of the OFC patient and other craniofacial anomalies is widely regarded as a multi-/ interdisciplinary enterprise that begins even in the prenatal stage with family counseling and continues days after birth, extending throughout life. The average lifetime medical cost per child with orofacial cleft is significant, at $100,000 [19]. One of the goals of the treatment of patients with OFC is to obtain good dental arch relationship and adequate facial growth associated with esthetically pleasing face and good speech. For achieving these goals, it is important to recognize that care of the patient with OFC is complex, involving multiple health-care providers, care coordinators, institutions, services, and other agencies. Traditionally, the treatment of OFC patients has relied upon craniofacial and cleft teams or centers, sometimes working in coordination with private practitioners. These centers provide a coordinated, inter-/multidisciplinary approach generally including experienced and qualified physicians and health-care profession-als from different specialties, such as surgical (plastic and maxillofacial surgeons), ENT, pediatric and general dentists, orthodontists, prosthodontists, speech therapists, psychologists, social workers, and allied health disciplines. Teams have become the standard in assessment and treatment of children with craniofacial anomalies like OFC [20–24]. The role of dentistry in treating individuals with cleft and craniofacial anomalies is the comprehensive preventative and therapeutic oral health care.

Prenatal diagnosis can be performed at 13–14 weeks of gestation when the soft tissues of the fetal face can be visualized sonographically [25]. Ideally, coronal view and axial planes are optimal for visualization of the fetal lip and palate in ultrasound images [26, 27]. Three-dimensional ultrasound [28, 29] and magnetic resonance imaging [30] also can provide a clear image of the malformation and may enhance detection of isolated cleft palate. Prenatal diagnosis of cleft lip and palate is a reality today, and in cases of labial clefts detected during prenatal period, parents can be

psychologically prepared before the birth of the child. Not only technical preparation regarding the birth but also a moral and social preparation of the family and friends for the reception of a child with an OFC can be arranged. Prenatal preparation of the parents and family support group can help promote earlier acceptance of a child with a craniofacial malformation [26] (Fig. 8.1).

Management of Newborns with OFC

Immediately after birth, feeding instructions, counseling, diagnosis by a geneticist, and a pediatric consultation should be arranged for the family. The newborn will need a hearing test while in the hospital, and assessment of the cleft is also provided. In the case of wide clefts, lip taping can start immediately [31, 32] The American Cleft Palate-Craniofacial Association advocates cleft repair by 18 months in a normally developing infant [20]. The timing of palatal repair must consider the potential for speech delay if the repair

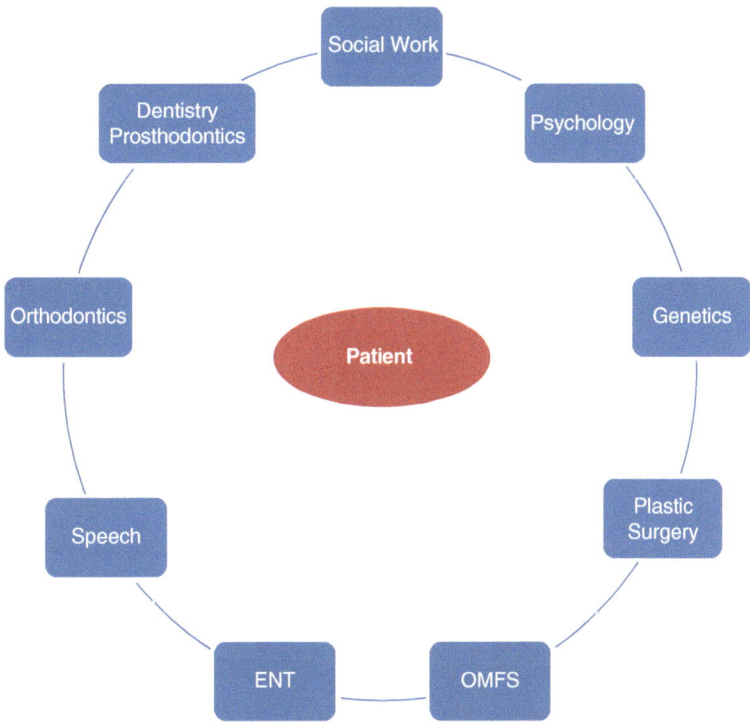

Fig. 8.1 Scheme of the professional structure of a multi-/interdisciplinary craniofacial team

is performed too late against the possible interference with normal craniofacial growth if performed too early. Certain centers support earlier repair to reduce the risk of velopharyngeal insufficiency, which has been shown to increase by 6 % for each month the repair is delayed beyond 7 months [33]. Surgical repair is a critical, time-sensitive event early in the care of patients with cleft palate; palatal integrity is essential during the key periods of speech development [34]. Parents of infants with OFC should begin discussions with a pediatric dentist to provide parental information and support; develop a strategy of caries prevention, growth, and development monitoring; and consider a referral to an orthodontist for presurgical infant orthopedics (e.g., nasal alveolar molding, NAM) when appropriate.

Nasal Alveolar Molding (NAM)

Nasal alveolar molding (NAM) is increasingly being used for treatment of orofacial cleft nose deformity before primary repair [35]. Nasal alveolar molding is used effectively to enable tension-free reconstruction of cleft lips and reshape the nasal cartilage and mold the maxillary arch before cleft lip repair and primary rhinoplasty. It provides esthetic and functional benefits of nasal tip and alar symmetry and improved dental arch form [35–37]. The conventional NAM protocol includes alignment and approximation of the alveolar segments, repositioning deformed nasal cartilages, effective retraction of the protruded premaxilla, and

lengthening of the deficient columella to achieve surgical soft tissue repair under minimal tension, with optimal conditions for minimal scar formation and increased nose symmetry [35–43]. NAM has significantly enhanced the ability of the interdisciplinary team to improve and maintain adequate nasolabial esthetics after the primary lip/nasal surgery in children with orofacial clefts. Infants are evaluated as early as possible, ideally within the first 2 weeks of life.

After the infant is examined to investigate whether any respiratory difficulties exist and to ensure that he/she is in good general health, the orthodontist/dentist takes an impression of the maxillary arch using an impression tray of acrylic resin that is slightly larger than the maxillary arch (Fig. 8.2). This is chosen from a collection of variously sized trays made from previously obtained maxillary dental casts. After the impression is taken, a stone cast is obtained from the impression and duplicated. The original cast is preserved for the patient record, and the second cast is used for fabrication of the appliance. A palatal plate is made of light-cured or thermo-cured resin, and the modified nasal stent is then added to the plate [35, 44, 45]. On the delivery appointment, the appliance is fit to the maxillary arch; a retentive loop is placed at the distal end of the wire; and a small piece of light-cured resin is cured to the tip of the nasal stent. Once the appliance is adjusted, the parents or guardians are given detailed oral and written instructions for placement, removal, and care of the appliance. They are also instructed to look for signs of irritation caused by the prosthesis. The appliance is retained with denture paste adhesive.

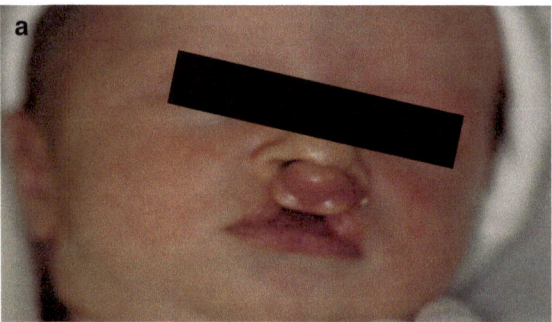 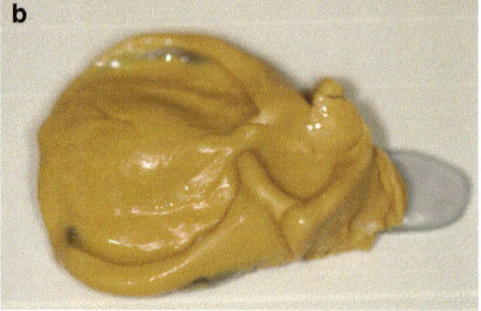

Fig. 8.2 (**a**) A 2-week old child with bilateral complete cleft lip and palate. (**b**) Impression in preparation for NAM

The patients are followed weekly for adjustments; nasal and alveolar moldings are initiated at the same time. Adjustments are made to improve comfort, guide alveolar segments' reposition, and readjust the molding pressure on the nasal cartilage. The goals are, initially, to lengthen the deficient columella and to reposition the apex of the alar cartilages toward the tip of the nose and, later, to maintain the achieved morphologic changes. The appliance is worn continuously except for cleaning after feeding until cleft lip surgery is performed, usually at age 3 or 4 months. Timing for surgery may be guided by the progress of nasal and alveolar molding [46].

Management of Toddlers and Preschool Children with OFC

OFC children often experience issues with feeding, swallowing, esthetics, and poor oral health [47, 48]. *The American Academy of Pediatric Dentistry* recommends that during this period, it is important to inform parents and/or guardians how important it is to establish a dental home for all infants, children, adolescents, and persons with special health-care needs. Establishing the dental home is initiated by the identification and interaction of caregivers and family members, resulting in a heightened awareness of all issues impacting the patient's oral health.

It is recommended to establish a dental home when the first primary tooth erupts in the mouth or within the first year of age. Ideally, parents should contact a dental clinic where comprehensive, continuously accessible, family-centered, coordinated, compassionate, and culturally effective care is available and delivered or supervised by qualified child health specialists. Preventative strategies can be implemented at this period with oral hygiene instructions, diet counseling, and application of fluoride varnish. The water source also needs to be evaluated (well or city water) to assure ideal levels of fluoride in water. Fluoridated tooth paste can also be used, but in a limited amount (a grain rice size smear until 3 years of age) so the child will experience the benefits of

fluoride in dental caries prevention with a reduced risk of enamel damage due to dental fluorosis [49, 50]. Limitation in frequency and sugar-based food intake is very important to reduce the risk of developing dental caries [51]. It is recommended that until 6 years of age, sweet milk (such as chocolate milk), sodas, and juices should be limited to no more than 4 oz per day, and ideally children should drink these beverages at main meals and have their teeth clean afterwards.

In summary, pediatric dentists would continue working with strategies for preventing dental caries, diet counseling, perioperative care, infant orthopedics when indicated, and growth and development monitoring and provide surgical and restorative care if necessary.

Tooth Development in the Cleft Region

Subjects with OFC have been found to have a higher prevalence of dental anomalies, such as variations in tooth number and position and reduced tooth dimensions, predominantly localized in the area of the cleft defect [52–54]. Also, a higher prevalence of enamel discoloration in children with OFC has been found when compared with a normal control group; this defect has been mainly attributed to trauma at the time of cleft surgery [55]. Hypodontia of the cleft-side permanent lateral incisor (49.8 %) and delayed root development in comparison with the contralateral tooth are also common issues reported in OFC subjects [53]. Therefore, the dentists should explain to parents and guardians the potential problems associated with missing teeth and the orthodontic/prosthetic possibilities for habilitation in the future.

Management of School Children with OFC

In addition to anticipatory guidance and preventative care already provided at preschool age, pediatric dentists will provide surgical and restorative care for OFC children as needed. Children with clefts are at a significant risk for caries of the primary incisors [56]. The prevalence of dental caries in the deciduous dentition was found to be greater in a group of children with OFC compared to children with OFC [57].

Children in the mixed dentition should be evaluated for determining optimal timing for secondary alveolar bone grafting. Patients with cleft lip and palate have a bony deficiency in the tooth-bearing alveolar region of the palate. To repair this bony deficiency, secondary alveolar bone grafting is carried out to provide adequate periodontal and bony support in to which the canine can erupt [58]. The ideal time for performing alveolar bone grafting in patients with OFC varies. However, grafting is highly successful in subjects with age ranging from 9 to 12 years and when the canine root is one fourth to one half formed, which means, before canine eruption [59, 60]. After surgery, canines in the cleft area will present normal root development in most cases with spontaneous eruption through autogenous bone grafting. Also, it can be expected that the canines may erupt more slowly through the bone graft, and in some cases surgical and/or orthodontic intervention (exposure and bonding) will be required to complete eruption.

In patients with bilateral cleft lip and palate, the premaxilla projects itself up and forward in various degrees because it is separated from the maxillary processes, which can be collapsed or distant from each other. The teeth adjacent to the cleft can present a deficiency in the alveolar bone thickness and height, restricting the possibilities of orthodontic treatment. Depsit these developmental deficiencies and issues the teeth adjacent to the cleft often present with good periodontal bone support during the stage of mixed dentition [59, 61–63]. Buccal and mesiodistal orthodontic movement as well as rotational movements of maxillary anterior teeth before alveolar bone graft should be avoided or carefully conducted in these patients [63, 64].

Speech remains a critical consideration: when surgical correction is not an option or has to be delayed for medical reasons or by parent's choice, then appliances can be fabricate to help with speech. Although surgery is the most frequently chosen approach for improving velopharyngeal function, a prosthetic device can be an option for some patients. These appliances are fabricated to be placed in the mouth, like an orthodontic retainer. Basically there are two types of speech appliances for children: the speech bulb and the palatal lift. When patients present with short palate, the speech bulb can be fabricated to partially close off the space between the soft palate and the throat [65, 66]. When there is inadequate palatal muscle function, even with appropriate palatal length, the palatal lift appliance can serve to lift the soft palate to a position that makes palatal closure possible [67]. It is recommended that prosthetic appliances be fabricated for children at least 5 years of age, and parents should closely supervise the use of these appliances [68, 69]. Children with submucous cleft palates (SMCPs) frequently suffer from delayed diagnosis that can result in poor speech outcomes. Furthermore, variability in the clinical severity of SMCPs can make treatment decisions challenging. Studies have established magnetic resonance imaging (MRI) as a reliable method to identify abnormalities in velopharyngeal muscle position, information that has potential to assist with treatment decisions (Fig. 8.3).

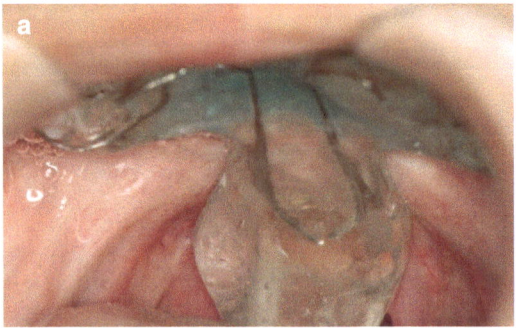 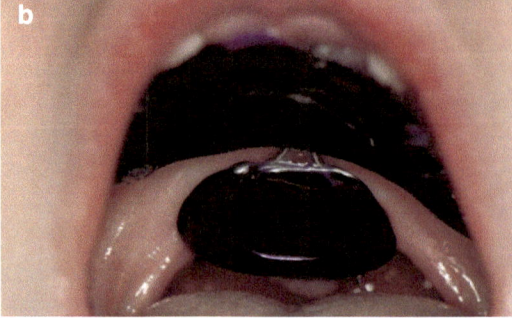

Fig. 8.3 (**a**) Palatal obturator in an 8-year-old child with short soft palate. Family would like to postpone surgical correction. (**b**) Palatal lift appliance of a 7-year-old child, appliance is used to help in elevating the palate to achieve palatal closure and reduce nasal air leakage

The pediatric dentist should work in coordination with orthodontists and oral maxillofacial surgeons in preparation for alveolar bone graft when necessary. They also will work with speech pathologists when a speech appliance is recommended and continue with measures for preventing dental caries and surgically remove primary teeth in surgical sites when indicated.

Management of Adolescents with OFC

Optimal management of patients with OFC is a continuous challenge. The surgical and clinical procedures carried out during infancy and childhood aim to create a foundation for development of normal speech, improvement of facial appearance, establishment of functional occlusion, and to strengthen self-esteem. However, there are reports showing that these early interventions can result in maxillary growth restriction that produce secondary deformities of the jaw and malocclusion, which also affect speech and self-esteem [70].

Adolescents with OFC not only have to deal with the developmental changes that naturally occur at this age, but also they must cope with special concerns common to their chronic condition such as: integrating their facial differences into an already changing body image, establishing interpersonal relationships despite possible dissatisfaction with facial appearance, relating to medical staff as young adults rather than children, and coping with surgeries that can alter and improve their facial appearance, but probably will not eliminate facial scarring.

Adolescents commonly recieve orthodontic treatment for alignment of their teeth and optimizing their occlusion. Additionally, they can have orthodontic treatment in preparation for orthognathic surgery that will occur at skeletal maturity. Orthognathic surgery is used to treat patients with cleft lip and palate who have a large skeletal class III malocclusion with variable degrees of anteroposterior, vertical, and transverse maxillary growth deficiency. Therefore, many of these patients will need orthognathic surgery at late teenage years when pubertal growth is complete.

During this phase, pediatric dentists and or general dentists have an important role in preventing dental caries and gingival inflammation by providing professional cleaning and oral hygiene instructions to the adolescents and their parents or guardians. Also, restorative treatment might be needed in cavitated caries lesions or in some cases for esthetic modifications of anterior teeth with resin composite direct restorations.

When implant-supported prosthetic rehabilitation is planned, the general dentist will need to refer the patient to a periodontist or oral maxillofacial surgeon for a regraft of the cleft area and implant placement and may refer to a prosthodontists for final oral habilitation [71, 72].

Management of Adults with OFC

There are still some adult patients with unrepaired OFC who will require oral care. Most of these individuals did not have a chance to have their clefts repaired surgically, or they presented with large clefts that could not be completely correct with surgical procedures, resulting in residual oronasal fistulas. Many of these patients are adults or elderly, and at their younger ages, there was no surgical alternative for repair, or they did not have access to proper care during childhood. In addition, they may have missing permanent teeth, deformed teeth, or even supernumerary teeth in the cleft area. Some patients reach adolescence or adulthood with unrepaired oronasal fistulas and alveolar clefts (bone discontinuity defects in the alveolus), even though the primary cleft defect has been repaired. The severity of residual deformities of the repaired cleft lip and nose may contribute to functional (mainly speech) and esthetic concerns. In adolescents and adults who have undergone cleft defect repair, common consequences include anterior and posterior crossbites; midface hypoplasia; anteroposterior, vertical, and transverse maxillary deficiency; residual lip and nasal deformities; and speech problems [73, 74].

Since orthognathic surgery (corrective jaw surgery) can affect significantly affect facial growth and development in patients with cleft lip and palate, end-stage reconstruction should be considered when these patients have reached skeletal maturity, which is usually age 15 years for females and 16–18 years or older for males [75–77]. If surgery is performed prior to completion of facial growth, the adverse effect on maxillary growth and continued growth of the mandible can result in recurrence of the facial deformity and malocclusion [76, 77]. In some cases, for esthetic and psychosocial reasons, surgery can be done at an earlier age with the understanding that it may need to be repeated after growth is complete [78–80].

Prosthetic Reconstruction

Adult patients who did not receive proper treatment for cleft palate are challenging for clinicians in terms of prosthetic rehabilitation. Moreover, during the late stages of adulthood when patients become edentulous, prosthetic reconstruction becomes even more challenging [81, 82]. Prosthetic rehabilitation requires adequate hard and soft tissue support. This aspect is of particular importance when the relationship of various anatomic structures is considered after reconstructive surgery [83, 84].

Patients who did not receive proper treatment for OFC often have several disorders such as: immature and collapsed maxillary arch, dysphagia, hypernasal speech, compromised chewing ability, palate with scar tissue, resorbed alveolar ridges, loss of vestibular depth, and oronasal fistulas. In addition, during the later stages of life when patients become edentulous, those issues related with OFC become troubling and more challenging in terms of prosthetic rehabilitation [81, 84].

Alveolar clefts are frequently associated with missing teeth [85, 86]. Management of the cleft after grafting involves either eruption of the canine in substitution for the missing tooth or tooth replacement using prosthetic means. Prosthetic methods include removable prosthesis, a fixed dental prosthesis (FDP), or a single tooth dental implant. The basic objectives of prosthodontic therapy include providing a comfortable, esthetically acceptable prosthesis that restores the impaired physiologic activities of speech, deglutition, mastication, and occlusion and preserving the remaining teeth and tissue [87].

Palatal Obturator

A residual oronasal communication (fistula) may be present even after surgical correction of the cleft in some cases. When that occurs, either on the palate or in the alveolar ridge or labial vestibule, they can result in speech, with undesirable nasal air emission or contribute to compromised articulation [88]. The main goal of a palatal obturator is to cover the fistula, to improve speech. Most of the time, it reduces hypernasality and corrects compensatory articulations.

The obturator can be used as a temporary appliance, while surgical correction is not possible or in some adult patients as a definitive prosthodontic appliance. As a temporary appliance, the obturator can be fabricated with resin acrylic, and it will cover the palate (palatal plate), and the retention is obtained with clasps fabricated with orthodontic wire. Most of the time, in those cases, the design will be similar to an orthodontic retainer.

However, in adult patients, when surgical correction is not an alternative, the prosthodontic obturator can be fabricated following the same principles applied for the fabrication of removable partial prostheses, with the metal infrastructure been fabricated with titanium or Co-Cr alloy [89] (Fig. 8.4). Removable prostheses are commonly indicated when clefts were not surgically closed, for oronasal fistula closure, and when a speech appliance is indicated [90, 91].

Fixed dental prostheses (FDPs) have an historic basis, but present many limitations for managing OFC patients. A small cohort treated using FDP ($n = 18$) revealed no patients with failed teeth but a 22 % complication rate over an extended observation period (7.4–24.9 years). The authors contend that local conditions render implant placement difficult and conventional FDP therapy remains the treatment of choice. However, esthetic parameters and patient-reported outcomes were not defined [92].

While dental implants and three-unit FDPs share similar 10-year survival rates [93], the use of an FDP for the OFC patient requires a more complex FDP involving more teeth. Complex FDPs do not enjoy equally high survival rates and suffer far greater complications [94]. Endosseous dental implant therapy does not involve destruction of

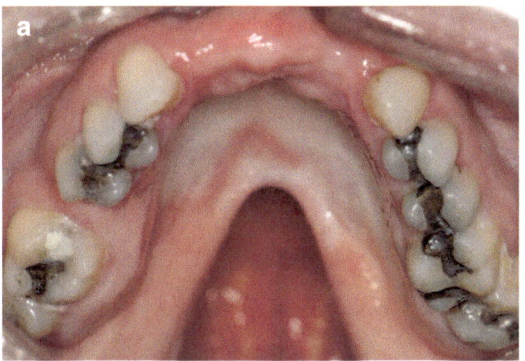
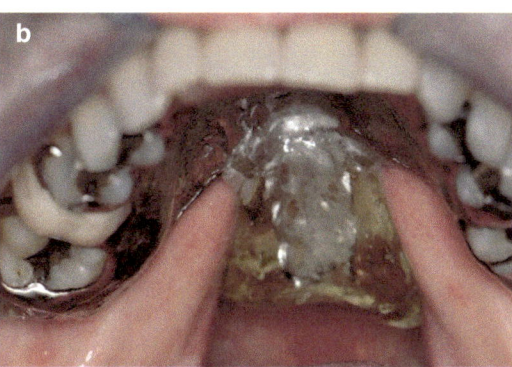

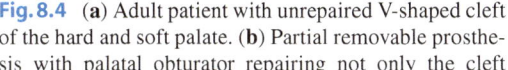

Fig. 8.4 (**a**) Adult patient with unrepaired V-shaped cleft of the hard and soft palate. (**b**) Partial removable prosthesis with palatal obturator repairing not only the cleft palate as well as missing teeth, resulting in functional and esthetic rehabilitation

adjacent teeth for a fixed dental prosthesis (FDP) or involvement of removable prostheses. A single dental implant eliminates destruction of adjacent teeth for FDPs, potentially avoiding the greater risks reported for the larger FDP. Further, the use of FDPs without attendant regrafting of the alveolus is possible, but fails to structurally address the underlying tissue deficiency that support lip, alar, and general facial architecture.

Dental implants have been used for tooth replacement in OFC patients [95], but truly comprehensive assessments of this therapy have not been reported. Prospective studies of dental implant outcomes in OFC patients have typically involved fewer than 50 subjects and examined implant survival only general terms such as patient age, gender, and the type of cleft.

Future Directions

With the development of new technologies for early diagnosis of craniofacial anomalies, families could be informed about the orofacial cleft before birth. Molecular genetics advances and evaluation of families around the world have led to identification of the causative genes of numerous syndromes and conditions involving OFCs (e.g., Van der Woude syndrome OMIM #119300, ectrodactyly, ectodermal dysplasia cleft syndrome OMIM #129900). While high-resolution 2D scanning remains the cornerstone of prenatal diagnosis, new 3D approaches continue to expand our ability to assess the craniofacial complex and clefts prenatally with great accuracy than ever before. Early diagnosis allows parents, family members, and their friends to be better oriented about the management of orofacial clefts regarding the steps to be followed and the potential costs involved for therapy to adulthood. In addition, parents can be in contact with other families of children born with orofacial cleft to develop a network of support [96, 97].

Adjunctive therapeutic strategies based on tissue engineering are being developed that will improve soft surgical outcomes such as bone augmentation and muscle development to enhance palate function. New intervention methods for cleft repair using stem cells could bring new alternative treatments in the future [98]. However, the most important aspect of the treatment of children born with orofacial cleft is to provide comprehensive care that can be effectively provided by craniofacial teams. Cleft and craniofacial teams are widely seen as an effective mean to avoid fragmentation and dehumanization in the delivery of highly specialized health care [99–101].

References

1. Grosen D, et al. A cohort study of recurrence patterns among more than 54,000 relatives of oral cleft cases in Denmark: support for the multifactorial threshold model of inheritance. J Med Genet. 2010;47(3):162–8.

2. Mangold E, et al. Genome-wide association study identifies two susceptibility loci for nonsyndromic cleft lip with or without cleft palate. Nat Genet. 2010;42(1):24–6.

3. Seto-Salvia N, Stanier P. Genetics of cleft lip and/or cleft palate: association with other common anomalies. Eur J Med Genet. 2014;57(8):381–93.

4. Doray B, et al. Epidemiology of orofacial clefts (1995–2006) in France (Congenital Malformations of Alsace Registry). Arch Pediatr. 2012;19(10):1021–9.

5. Coleman Jr JR, Sykes JM. The embryology, classification, epidemiology, and genetics of facial clefting. Facial Plast Surg Clin North Am. 2001;9(1):1–13.

6. Parker SE, et al. Updated National Birth Prevalence estimates for selected birth defects in the United States, 2004–2006. Birth Defects Res A Clin Mol Teratol. 2010;88(12):1008–16.

7. Wangsrimongkol T, et al. Prevalence and types of dental anomaly in a Thai non-syndromic oral cleft sample. J Med Assoc Thai. 2013;96 Suppl 4:S25–35.

8. Kalaskar R, et al. Prevalence and evaluation of environmental risk factors associated with cleft lip and palate in a central Indian population. Pediatr Dent. 2013;35(3):279–83.

9. Amaratunga AN, Chandrasekera A. Incidence of cleft lip and palate in Sri Lanka. J Oral Maxillofac Surg. 1989;47(6):559–61.

10. Hashmi SS, et al. Prevalence of nonsyndromic oral clefts in Texas: 1995–1999. Am J Med Genet A. 2005;134(4):368–72.

11. Tolarova MM, Cervenka J. Classification and birth prevalence of orofacial clefts. Am J Med Genet. 1998;75(2):126–37.

12. DeRoo LA, Gaudino JA, Edmonds LD. Orofacial cleft malformations: associations with maternal and infant characteristics in Washington State. Birth Defects Res A Clin Mol Teratol. 2003;67(9):637–42.

13. Khoury MJ, Erickson JD, James LM. Maternal factors in cleft lip with or without palate: evidence from interracial crosses in the United States. Teratology. 1983;27(3):351–7.

14. Shaw GM, Croen LA, Curry CJ. Isolated oral cleft malformations: associations with maternal and infant characteristics in a California population. Teratology. 1991;43(3):225–8.

15. Leite IC, Koifman S. Oral clefts, consanguinity, parental tobacco and alcohol use: a case-control study in Rio de Janeiro. Braz Oral Res. 2009;23(1):31–7.

16. Lammer EJ, et al. Maternal smoking, genetic variation of glutathione s-transferases, and risk for orofacial clefts. Epidemiology. 2005;16(5):698–701.

17. Jia ZL, et al. Maternal malnutrition, environmental exposure during pregnancy and the risk of non-syndromic orofacial clefts. Oral Dis. 2011; 17(6):584–9.

18. Liau JY, Sadove AM, van Aalst JA. An evidence-based approach to cleft palate repair. Plast Reconstr Surg. 2010;126(6):2216–21.

19. Basseri B, et al. Current national incidence, trends, and health care resource utilization of cleft lip-cleft palate. Plast Reconstr Surg. 2011;127(3):1255–62.

20. Parameters for evaluation and treatment of patients with cleft lip/palate or other craniofacial anomalies. American Cleft Palate-Craniofacial Association. March, 1993. Cleft Palate Craniofac J. 1993;30 Suppl:S1–16.

21. Sharp HM. Ethical decision-making in interdisciplinary team care. Cleft Palate Craniofac J. 1995;32(6):495–9.

22. Strauss RP, et al. Physicians and the communication of "bad news": parent experiences of being informed of their child's cleft lip and/or palate. Pediatrics. 1995;96(1 Pt 1):82–9.

23. Strauss RP. Cleft palate and craniofacial teams in the United States and Canada: a national survey of team organization and standards of care. The American Cleft Palate-Craniofacial Association (ACPA) Team Standards Committee. Cleft Palate Craniofac J. 1998;35(6):473–80.

24. Grosse SD, et al. Models of comprehensive multidisciplinary care for individuals in the United States with genetic disorders. Pediatrics. 2009;123(1):407–12.

25. Franco D, et al. The importance of pre-natal diagnosis of facial congenital malformations. J Plast Reconstr Aesthet Surg. 2013;66(8):e236–7.

26. Amstalden-Mendes LG, et al. Time of diagnosis of oral clefts: a multicenter study. J Pediatr (Rio J). 2011;87(3):225–30.

27. Sommerlad M, et al. Detection of lip, alveolar ridge and hard palate abnormalities using two-dimensional ultrasound enhanced with the three-dimensional reverse-face view. Ultrasound Obstet Gynecol. 2010;36(5):596–600.

28. Platt LD, Devore GR, Pretorius DH. Improving cleft palate/cleft lip antenatal diagnosis by 3-dimensional sonography: the "flipped face" view. J Ultrasound Med. 2006;25(11):1423–30.

29. McGahan MC, et al. Multislice display of the fetal face using 3-dimensional ultrasonography. J Ultrasound Med. 2008;27(11):1573–81.

30. Mailath-Pokorny M, et al. What does magnetic resonance imaging add to the prenatal ultrasound diagnosis of facial clefts? Ultrasound Obstet Gynecol. 2010;36(4):445–51.

31. Vargervik K, Oberoi S, Hoffman WY. Team care for the patient with cleft: UCSF protocols and outcomes. J Craniofac Surg. 2009;20 Suppl 2:1668–71.

32. Cassell CH, Daniels J, Meyer RE. Timeliness of primary cleft lip/palate surgery. Cleft Palate Craniofac J. 2009;46(6):588–97.

33. Sullivan SR, et al. Palatoplasty outcomes in nonsyndromic patients with cleft palate: a 29-year assessment of one surgeon's experience. J Craniofac Surg. 2009;20 Suppl 1:612–6.

34. Abbott MM, Kokorowski PJ, Meara JG. Timeliness of surgical care in children with special health care needs: delayed palate repair for publicly insured and

minority children with cleft palate. J Pediatr Surg. 2011;46(7):1319–24.

35. Santiago PE, et al. Reduced need for alveolar bone grafting by presurgical orthopedics and primary gingivoperiosteoplasty. Cleft Palate Craniofac J. 1998;35(1):77–80.

36. Cutting C, et al. Presurgical columellar elongation and primary retrograde nasal reconstruction in one-stage bilateral cleft lip and nose repair. Plast Reconstr Surg. 1998;101(3):630–9.

37. Cutting C, Grayson B, Brecht L. Columellar elongation in bilateral cleft lip. Plast Reconstr Surg. 1998;102(5):1761–2.

38. Gateno J, et al. A new Le Fort I internal distraction device in the treatment of severe maxillary hypoplasia. J Oral Maxillofac Surg. 2005;63(1):148–54.

39. Singh GD, Levy-Bercowski D, Santiago PE. Three-dimensional nasal changes following nasoalveolar molding in patients with unilateral cleft lip and palate: geometric morphometrics. Cleft Palate Craniofac J. 2005;42(4):403–9.

40. Spengler AL, et al. Presurgical nasoalveolar molding therapy for the treatment of bilateral cleft lip and palate: a preliminary study. Cleft Palate Craniofac J. 2006;43(3):321–8.

41. Ezzat CF, et al. Presurgical nasoalveolar molding therapy for the treatment of unilateral cleft lip and palate: a preliminary study. Cleft Palate Craniofac J. 2007;44(1):8–12.

42. Singh GD, et al. Three-dimensional facial morphology following surgical repair of unilateral cleft lip and palate in patients after nasoalveolar molding. Orthod Craniofac Res. 2007;10(3):161–6.

43. Santiago PE, Schuster LA, Levy-Bercowski D. Management of the alveolar cleft. Clin Plast Surg. 2014;41(2):219–32.

44. Maull DJ, et al. Long-term effects of nasoalveolar molding on three-dimensional nasal shape in unilateral clefts. Cleft Palate Craniofac J. 1999;36(5):391–7.

45. Grayson BH, Maull D. Nasoalveolar molding for infants born with clefts of the lip, alveolus, and palate. Clin Plast Surg. 2004;31(2):149–58, vii.

46. Da Silveira AC, et al. Modified nasal alveolar molding appliance for management of cleft lip defect. J Craniofac Surg. 2003;14(5):700–3.

47. Parapanisiou V, et al. Oral health status and behaviour of Greek patients with cleft lip and palate. Eur Arch Paediatr Dent. 2009;10(2):85–9.

48. Miller CK. Feeding issues and interventions in infants and children with clefts and craniofacial syndromes. Semin Speech Lang. 2011;32(2):115–26.

49. Ramos-Gomez FJ, et al. Minimal intervention dentistry: part 3. Paediatric dental care–prevention and management protocols using caries risk assessment for infants and young children. Br Dent J. 2012;213(10):501–8.

50. Crall JJ. Development and integration of oral health services for preschool-age children. Pediatr Dent. 2005;27(4):323–30.

51. Barbers BC, Rojas AC. Effects of combined tooth-brushing and sweet diet limitation in dental caries prevention in a school setting after two-and-a-half years. J Philipp Dent Assoc. 1986;36(1):3–9.

52. Haring FN. Dental development in cleft and noncleft subjects. Angle Orthod. 1976;46(1):47–50.

53. Ribeiro LL, et al. Dental development of permanent lateral incisor in complete unilateral cleft lip and palate. Cleft Palate Craniofac J. 2002;39(2):193–6.

54. Qureshi WA, Beiraghi S, Leon-Salazar V. Dental anomalies associated with unilateral and bilateral cleft lip and palate. J Dent Child (Chic). 2012;79(2):69–73.

55. Lucas VS, et al. Dental health indices and caries associated microflora in children with unilateral cleft lip and palate. Cleft Palate Craniofac J. 2000;37(5):447–52.

56. Johnsen DC, Dixon M. Dental caries of primary incisors in children with cleft lip and palate. Cleft Palate J. 1984;21(2):104–9.

57. Bokhout B, et al. Incidence of dental caries in the primary dentition in children with a cleft lip and/or palate. Caries Res. 1997;31(1):8–12.

58. Helms JA, Speidel TM, Denis KL. Effect of timing on long-term clinical success of alveolar cleft bone grafts. Am J Orthod Dentofacial Orthop. 1987;92(3):232–40.

59. Troxell JB, Fonseca RJ, Osbon DB. A retrospective study of alveolar cleft grafting. J Oral Maxillofac Surg. 1982;40(11):721–5.

60. El Deeb M, et al. Canine eruption into grafted bone in maxillary alveolar cleft defects. Cleft Palate J. 1982;19(1):9–16.

61. Sharma S, et al. Secondary alveolar bone grafting: radiographic and clinical evaluation. Ann Maxillofac Surg. 2012;2(1):41–5.

62. Nwoku AL, et al. Retrospective analysis of secondary alveolar cleft grafts using iliac of chin bone. J Craniofac Surg. 2005;16(5):864–8.

63. Dewinter G, et al. Dental abnormalities, bone graft quality, and periodontal conditions in patients with unilateral cleft lip and palate at different phases of orthodontic treatment. Cleft Palate Craniofac J. 2003;40(4):343–50.

64. Semb G, Ramstad T. The influence of alveolar bone grafting on the orthodontic and prosthodontic treatment of patients with cleft lip and palate. Dent Update. 1999;26(2):60–4.

65. Rosen MS, Bzoch KR. The prosthetic speech appliance in rehabilitation of patients with cleft palate. J Am Dent Assoc. 1958;57(2):203–10.

66. Tachimura T, Nohara K, Wada T. Effect of placement of a speech appliance on levator veli palatini muscle activity during speech. Cleft Palate Craniofac J. 2000;37(5):478–82.

67. Raju H, Padmanabhan TV, Narayan A. Effect of a palatal lift prosthesis in individuals with velopharyngeal incompetence. Int J Prosthodont. 2009;22(6):579–85.

68. Raj N, Raj V, Aeran H. Interim palatal lift prosthesis as a constituent of multidisciplinary approach in the treatment of velopharyngeal incompetence. J Adv Prosthodont. 2012;4(4):243–7.

69. Premkumar S. Clinical application of palatal lift appliance in velopharyngeal incompetence. J Indian Soc Pedod Prev Dent. 2011;29(6 Suppl 2):S70–3.

70. Ross RB. Treatment variables affecting facial growth in complete unilateral cleft lip and palate. Cleft Palate J. 1987;24(1):5–77.

71. de Barros Ferreira Jr S, et al. Survival of dental implants in the cleft area – a retrospective study. Cleft Palate Craniofac J. 2010;47(6):586–90.

72. Wermker K, et al. Dental implants in cleft lip, alveolus, and palate patients: a systematic review. Int J Oral Maxillofac Implants. 2014;29(2):384–90.

73. Shah CP, Wong D. Management of children with cleft lip and palate. Can Med Assoc J. 1980;122(1): 19–24.

74. Lin FH, Wang TC. Prosthodontic rehabilitation for edentulous patients with palatal defect: report of two cases. J Formos Med Assoc. 2011;110(2):120–4.

75. Siow KK, et al. Satisfaction of orthognathic surgical patients in a Malaysian population. J Oral Sci. 2002;44(3–4):165–71.

76. Wolford LM, et al. Orthognathic surgery in the young cleft patient: preliminary study on subsequent facial growth. J Oral Maxillofac Surg. 2008;66(12):2524–36.

77. Kumari P, et al. Stability of Cleft maxilla in Le Fort I Maxillary advancement. Ann Maxillofac Surg. 2013;3(2):139–43.

78. Bill J, et al. Orthognathic surgery in cleft patients. J Craniomaxillofac Surg. 2006;34 Suppl 2:77–81.

79. Waldron JM, et al. Cleft-affected children in Mayo: 1999–2007. J Ir Dent Assoc. 2011;57(6):316–8.

80. Meazzini MC, et al. Long-term follow-up of UCLP patients: surgical and orthodontic burden of care during growth and final orthognathic surgery need. Cleft Palate Craniofac J. 2013 Jul 23. [Epub ahead of print].

81. Guven O, et al. Surgical and prosthetic rehabilitation of edentulous adult cleft palate patients by dental implants. J Craniofac Surg. 2010;21(5):1538–41.

82. de Santis D, et al. Zygomatic and maxillary implants inserted by means of computer-assisted surgery in a patient with a cleft palate. J Craniofac Surg. 2010;21(3):858–62.

83. Guven O. Rehabilitation of severely atrophied mandible using free iliac crest bone grafts and dental implants: report of two cases. J Oral Implantol. 2007;33(3):122–6.

84. Laine J, et al. Rehabilitation of patients with congenital unrepaired cleft palate defects using free iliac crest bone grafts and dental implants. Int J Oral Maxillofac Implants. 2002;17(4):573–80.

85. Pegelow M, Alqadi N, Karsten AL. The prevalence of various dental characteristics in the primary and mixed dentition in patients born with non-syndromic unilateral cleft lip with or without cleft palate. Eur J Orthod. 2012;34(5):561–70.

86. Kuijpers MA, et al. Incidental findings on cone beam computed tomography scans in cleft lip and palate patients. Clin Oral Investig. 2014;18(4): 1237–44.

87. Devan MM. Biological demands of complete dentures. J Am Dent Assoc. 1952;45(5):524–7.

88. Murthy J, Sendhilnathan S, Hussain SA. Speech outcome following late primary palate repair. Cleft Palate Craniofac J. 2010;47(2):156–61.

89. Bridgeman JT, et al. Comparison of titanium and cobalt-chromium removable partial denture clasps. J Prosthet Dent. 1997;78(2):187–93.

90. Bartonova, et al. Long-term stability of prosthetic treatment of oronasal and oroantral communications. Acta Chir Plast. 2005;47(3):85–91.

91. Freitas JA, et al. Rehabilitative treatment of cleft lip and palate: experience of the Hospital for Rehabilitation of Craniofacial Anomalies/USP (HRAC/USP) – part 4: oral rehabilitation. J Appl Oral Sci. 2013;21(3):284–92.

92. Bidra AS. Esthetic and functional rehabilitation of a bilateral cleft palate patient with fixed prosthodontic therapy. J Esthet Restor Dent. 2012;24(4): 236–44.

93. Hochman N, et al. Functional and esthetic rehabilitation of an adolescent cleft lip and palate patient. Quintessence Int. 1991;22(5):401–4.

94. Krieger O, et al. Failures and complications in patients with birth defects restored with fixed dental prostheses and single crowns on teeth and/or implants. Clin Oral Implants Res. 2009;20(8):809–16.

95. Pjetursson BE, Lang NP. Prosthetic treatment planning on the basis of scientific evidence. J Oral Rehabil. 2008;35 Suppl 1:72–9.

96. Kaufman FL. Managing the cleft lip and palate patient. Pediatr Clin North Am. 1991;38(5): 1127–47.

97. Kuttenberger J, Ohmer JN, Polska E. Initial counselling for cleft lip and palate: parents' evaluation, needs and expectations. Int J Oral Maxillofac Surg. 2010;39(3):214–20.

98. Pourebrahim N, et al. A comparison of tissue-engineered bone from adipose-derived stem cell with autogenous bone repair in maxillary alveolar cleft model in dogs. Int J Oral Maxillofac Surg. 2013;42(5):562–8.

99. Gimbel M, et al. Repair of alveolar cleft defects: reduced morbidity with bone marrow stem cells in a resorbable matrix. J Craniofac Surg. 2007;18(4):895–901.

100. Strauss RP. The organization and delivery of craniofacial health services: the state of the art. Cleft Palate Craniofac J. 1999;36(3):189–95.

101. Matsuo A, et al. Osteogenic potential of cryopreserved human bone marrow-derived mesenchymal stem cells cultured with autologous serum. J Craniofac Surg. 2008;19(3):693–700.

Index